RURAL ONCOLOGY POCKET GUIDE

DR. MOHAMED ELGENDY, LMCC, CCFP, CANADA

ISBN:

978-1-997896-01-2 (eBook)
978-1-997896-02-9 (Paperback)
978-1-997896-03-6 (Hardcover)

DISCLAIMER

This pocket guide was developed with the assistance of advanced AI tools to streamline content generation. Every chapter has been thoroughly reviewed, edited, and authenticated by **Dr. Mohamed Elgendy, LMCC, CCFP (Canada)**, ensuring accuracy, credibility, and clinical authenticity. The result is a modern, innovative reference that blends the efficiency of AI with the rigor of professional medical expertise.

This booklet summarizes key oncology care principles and referral pathways derived from publicly available, evidence-based clinical resources. It does not reproduce proprietary algorithms, figures, or copyrighted material from subscription-only sources. The content is designed for educational purposes and quick clinical reference in rural and primary care settings; it is not a substitute for specialist consultation, institutional policies, or local oncology protocols.

Clinical responsibility remains with the treating physician. Always verify staging criteria, treatment options, and medication information with current product monographs, institutional references, and applicable regional standards before use in patient care.

ABOUT THE AUTHOR

Dr. Mohamed Elgendy is a licensed Canadian physician with the Licentiate of the Medical Council of Canada (LMCC) and Certification in Family Medicine (CCFP) from the College of Family Physicians of Canada. He has several years of hands-on experience as both a rural emergency physician and a family doctor, currently practicing in Saskatchewan, Canada. With a deep commitment to improving healthcare delivery in underserved communities, Dr. Elgendy focuses on practical, evidence-based medicine tailored to the realities of rural practice. His work bridges the gap between academic medicine and frontline care, offering accessible resources to help clinicians make confident, life-saving decisions in resource-limited settings

DEDICATION

This book is dedicated to the **patients in rural and remote communities** facing cancer with courage, faith, and resilience; to the **healthcare providers** who deliver oncology care with compassion, dedication, and ingenuity despite limited resources; and to my **family**, whose unwavering support and encouragement make every page of this work possible.

— Dr. Mohamed Elgendy

TABLE OF CONTENTS

PART A:
ONCOLOGY

CHAPTER 1:
Adrenal Lesion

1. Overview:

Adrenal lesions, also called adrenal incidentalomas, are increasingly detected due to widespread imaging.

While most are benign and nonfunctional, a small proportion represent hormonally active or malignant tumors.

The family physician in a rural setting plays an essential role in identifying red flags, ordering initial investigations, and arranging timely referral.

2. Initial Clinical Evaluation:

- **History:** Assess for symptoms of hormone excess — weight gain, hypertension, diabetes, hirsutism, muscle weakness, or paroxysmal headaches.
- **Physical Exam:** Measure blood pressure, check for Cushingoid features, virilization, or abdominal masses.
- **Review Medications:** Some drugs can alter cortisol or renin-aldosterone results.
- **Assess Cancer History:** Metastatic disease should be considered if the patient has a prior malignancy.

3. Hormonal Assessment:

Every adrenal lesion ≥1 cm warrants biochemical screening to exclude hormone excess:

- **Cortisol:** Overnight 1 mg dexamethasone suppression test.
- **Catecholamines:** Plasma free or urinary fractionated metanephrines to rule out pheochromocytoma.

- **Aldosterone/Renin Ratio:** For hypertensive or hypokalemic patients to assess for primary aldosteronism.
- **Androgens/Estrogens:** If virilization or feminization present.

These tests can usually be performed in rural hospitals or outpatient labs before referral.

4. Imaging Characteristics:

- **Benign Adenoma:** <4 cm, low attenuation (<10 HU on CT), homogeneous, smooth borders.
- **Suspicious Lesion:** ≥4 cm, irregular, heterogeneous, high attenuation (>20 HU), delayed washout, or calcifications.
- **MRI:** Can help differentiate adenoma from metastasis or carcinoma.
- **PET/CT:** Used in oncology patients to detect adrenal metastases.

5. Referral Criteria:

Urgent referral to endocrinology or oncology is indicated for:

- Functioning tumor (Cushing's, pheochromocytoma, hyperaldosteronism).
- Lesion ≥4 cm or growing >1 cm/year.
- Indeterminate imaging features.
- Known malignancy with new adrenal lesion.
- Tele-endocrinology consultation can assist rural physicians with work-up interpretation before transfer.

6. Role After Oncology Discharge:

After adrenalectomy or oncologic treatment, the rural family doctor provides follow-up, monitors hormone replacement, and detects recurrence or metastasis early.

Coordination with endocrinology and oncology ensures long-term safety and quality of life.

7. Post-Surgical and Hormonal Monitoring:

- **Adrenal Insufficiency:** Patients post-adrenalectomy may require hydrocortisone replacement; dose titrated under endocrinology guidance.
- **Blood Pressure and Electrolytes:** Regular monitoring for hypo/hypertension, hyponatremia, or hyperkalemia.
- **Hormone Testing:** Annual dexamethasone suppression or plasma metanephrine tests if initially functional.
- **Imaging:** Repeat CT or MRI every 6–12 months for 2 years, then as directed by oncology.

8. Managing Long-Term Complications:

- Cushing's or Addisonian Features: Adjust glucocorticoid replacement and provide stress-dose education.
- Pheochromocytoma Survivors: Lifelong blood pressure monitoring and catecholamine testing every 1–2 years.
- Metastatic Disease: Pain control, steroid replacement, and coordination with oncology or palliative care.
- The family physician ensures prompt recognition of hormonal imbalances and supports adherence to medications.

9. Health Promotion and Lifestyle:

- Encourage balanced diet, regular exercise, and weight management.
- Avoid excessive alcohol, caffeine, and smoking.
- Counsel on stress management and emergency steroid identification card use.
- Regular screening for diabetes, osteoporosis, and cardiovascular risk in post-Cushing's or steroid-treated patients.

CHAPTER 2:
Breast Cancer

1. Recognition and Screening

Early recognition and screening remain critical for improved survival. Family physicians are often the first contact in detection.

- Recognize red flags: new lump, nipple retraction, bloody or serous discharge, skin dimpling ('peau d'orange'), or non-resolving mastitis.
- Maintain low threshold for imaging in women over 30 or with risk factors.
- For men and elderly women, consider breast cancer even with atypical presentations.
- Offer mammography every 2 years for women aged 50–74 (CTFPHC guidelines).
- Discuss individualized screening for women 40–49 or high-risk groups (BRCA, family history, prior chest radiation).
- Encourage breast self-awareness, not formal self-exam, for early symptom reporting.
- Document findings thoroughly in EMR and schedule follow-up on all abnormal results.

2. Primary Care Diagnostic Approach

A systematic, evidence-based diagnostic process ensures timely referral and reduces missed diagnoses.

- Obtain comprehensive history: onset, duration, associated pain, discharge, family history, hormonal exposure, and previous imaging.
- Perform bilateral breast and axillary examination with patient seated and supine.

Imaging approach:

- <30 years: Ultrasound first-line.
- ≥30 years: Diagnostic mammogram and targeted ultrasound.
- Apply the Triple Test: Clinical exam + Imaging + Biopsy. If 2 out of 3 are suspicious, manage as malignant until proven otherwise.
- Order core needle biopsy for tissue confirmation; avoid FNA if possible for solid lesions.
- Baseline labs (CBC, LFTs, calcium, creatinine) if metastatic or systemic symptoms suspected.
- Ensure clear communication of results and next steps with the patient.
- Use tele-oncology or regional breast diagnostic programs where available.

3. Pre-Referral and Referral Workflow

Efficient coordination between primary care and oncology expedites diagnosis and treatment initiation.

Pre-Referral Management:

- Discuss results honestly and empathetically before referral.
- Review existing tests to prevent unnecessary duplication.
- Manage infection, pain, or anxiety as appropriate while awaiting referral.
- Coordinate tele-oncology consults for rural patients if oncology access is limited.
- Ensure EMR documentation includes exam findings, imaging, pathology, and labs.
- Confirm contact information and assist with travel documentation or appointment coordination.
- Arrange follow-up within 2–3 weeks to verify referral completion.

Referral Preparation:

- Urgent referral for palpable mass, BI-RADS ≥4, or nipple changes.
- Semi-urgent (2–4 weeks) for unresolved mastitis or indeterminate imaging.
- Routine referral for asymptomatic screening abnormalities.
- Include full clinical summary, pathology, and imaging reports; avoid repeat imaging within 6 months.
- Confirm receipt of referral and document communication in EMR.

4. Management, Complications, and Follow-Up

Although oncology teams direct treatment, the family physician's role continues throughout recovery and survivorship.

Treatment Overview (for patient discussion):

- Surgery – Lumpectomy or mastectomy ± axillary dissection.
- Radiation – To reduce local recurrence risk post-surgery.
- Chemotherapy – For aggressive or lymph node–positive disease.
- Endocrine therapy – Tamoxifen or aromatase inhibitors for ER/PR-positive cancers (5–10 years).
- Targeted therapy – Trastuzumab for HER2-positive disease.

Common Complications and Management in Primary Care:

- Lymphedema – Educate on limb positioning, compression sleeves, and physiotherapy.
- Cardiotoxicity – Monitor cardiac function for patients on anthracyclines or trastuzumab.
- Fatigue and anemia – Investigate and treat underlying causes (iron, B12, thyroid).

- Menopausal symptoms – Offer non-hormonal options (SSRIs, gabapentin) and lubricants as needed.
- Infection or wound issues – Provide wound care, antibiotics, or refer if severe.
- Psychological support – Screen for depression, anxiety, and address body image or sexual health concerns.

Follow-Up Schedule (Canadian guidelines):

- Years 1–3: every 3–6 months; Years 4–5: every 6–12 months; after 5 years: annually.
- Annual mammogram for any remaining breast tissue.
- Examine surgical site, nodes, and assess for recurrence (pain, cough, weight loss).
- Reinforce medication adherence and maintain continuity with oncology team.
- Encourage physical activity, smoking cessation, and healthy diet.
- Plan early palliative involvement if recurrence or advanced disease detected.

5. Family Doctor's Role in Ongoing Care – Q&A Scenario:

CASE: A 49-year-old woman presents with a firm, painless lump in her left breast for 3 weeks. No nipple discharge. No family history of cancer.

Q1. What are the first key steps in evaluation?

Perform full breast and axillary exam. Order diagnostic mammogram and ultrasound. Document all findings.

Q2. What investigations are needed next?

Request core needle biopsy for histologic diagnosis and baseline labs if systemic symptoms.

Q3. What is the likely diagnosis based on results?

Biopsy confirms invasive ductal carcinoma (IDC).

Q4. What should the family doctor do after diagnosis?

Explain diagnosis empathetically, provide written summary, and initiate oncology referral. Support patient emotionally and practically.

Q5. How should care continue post-treatment?

Provide post-surgery and survivorship follow-up focusing on wound care, lymphedema prevention, medication adherence, recurrence monitoring, and mental health support.

CHAPTER 3:
Cervical Cancer

1. Recognition and Screening:

- Cervical cancer is largely preventable through screening and HPV vaccination. Family physicians are key in early detection.
- Common symptoms: postcoital bleeding, intermenstrual bleeding, abnormal vaginal discharge, or pelvic pain.
- Advanced symptoms: pelvic mass, hematuria, rectal bleeding, or leg edema due to lymphatic obstruction.

Screening recommendations:

- Screen all individuals with a cervix aged 25–69 every 3 years with a Pap test (or every 5 years with HPV testing if available).
- Discontinue screening at age 70 if three consecutive negative results in the last 10 years.
- Immunocompromised or DES-exposed women: annual screening.
- Encourage HPV vaccination for all eligible individuals (both sexes) as primary prevention.
- Document last Pap/HPV test, sexual history, and HPV vaccination status in EMR.

2. Primary Care Diagnostic Approach:

- Family physicians often identify precancerous lesions or early cancers through screening and symptom evaluation.
- History: abnormal bleeding patterns, discharge, pelvic pain, sexual history, and prior Pap results.

- Physical exam: speculum exam for visible lesions, friable tissue, or contact bleeding; bimanual exam for masses or parametrial involvement.

Initial investigations:

- Pap smear or HPV test (if not up to date).
- STI testing (chlamydia, gonorrhea, trichomonas).
- Pregnancy test if reproductive age with abnormal bleeding.
- For visible suspicious lesion → do **not repeat Pap**; refer directly for colposcopy and biopsy.
- Imaging (pelvic ultrasound, MRI) guided by specialist if advanced disease suspected.

3. Pre-Referral and Referral Workflow

Pre-Referral Management:

- Manage anemia with iron or transfusion if severe before referral.
- Rule out and treat concurrent vaginal infections before biopsy or procedure.
- Counsel the patient regarding possible causes and emphasize the importance of timely specialist evaluation.
- Ensure up-to-date Pap and HPV results are available for referral package.
- Avoid performing cervical biopsy in primary care unless trained and resources for bleeding management are available.
- Provide emotional support and reassurance while arranging referral.

Referral Preparation:

Urgent referral for:

- Abnormal Pap showing high-grade lesion (HSIL, ASC-H, AGC).
- Visible cervical lesion with bleeding or ulceration.
- Postcoital or unexplained intermenstrual bleeding with suspicious findings.
- Semi-urgent referral (within 2–4 weeks) for low-grade abnormalities (LSIL) requiring colposcopy.
- Attach latest Pap/HPV results, relevant labs, and prior gynecologic history to referral letter.
- For remote/rural areas, arrange virtual consult or expedited travel support if access barriers exist.

4. Management, Complications, and Follow-Up

Family doctors play an ongoing role in patient education, follow-up, and survivorship care after oncology treatment.

Treatment Overview:

- Early-stage: cone biopsy, LEEP, or hysterectomy depending on lesion size and fertility goals.
- Locally advanced: chemoradiation (cisplatin-based).
- Metastatic or recurrent: systemic therapy (chemotherapy ± immunotherapy) or palliative radiotherapy.

Primary Care Role:

- Manage pain, anemia, and infection prophylaxis during treatment.
- Address vaginal dryness, dyspareunia, and urinary/bowel changes post-radiation.
- Provide emotional and psychosocial support for sexual health and fertility concerns.

- Reinforce adherence to follow-up schedules for recurrence detection.

Follow-Up Schedule:

- Every 3–6 months for the first 2 years, every 6–12 months for the next 3 years, then annually.
- Follow-up includes pelvic exam, Pap/HPV testing (if cervix retained), and symptom review.
- Refer promptly for new bleeding, pelvic pain, or discharge suggestive of recurrence.
- Encourage smoking cessation and healthy lifestyle.

5. Family Doctor's Role – Clinical Scenario (Q&A Format)

Case: A 36-year-old woman presents with postcoital bleeding for two months and a yellowish vaginal discharge. Her last Pap was 5 years ago.

Q1. What should be the first step in evaluation?

Perform a speculum exam to visualize the cervix, collect Pap and HPV samples, and rule out infection.

Q2. What findings warrant urgent referral?

A friable or ulcerated cervical lesion, or Pap results showing HSIL or carcinoma in situ.

Q3. What can be done before referral?

Treat any vaginal infection, manage anemia, and counsel regarding the importance of biopsy and follow-up.

Q4. What are common complications after treatment that family doctors manage?

Vaginal stenosis, menopausal symptoms, lymphedema, urinary frequency, and emotional distress.

Q5. How should follow-up be structured post-oncology discharge?

Pelvic exams every 3–6 months for two years, Pap/HPV testing as per oncology guidance, and prompt referral for recurrence symptoms.

CHAPTER 4:
Colon Cancer

1. Recognition and Screening:

- Colon cancer is often asymptomatic in early stages and may present during routine screening.
- Common symptoms: rectal bleeding, change in bowel habits, unexplained anemia, or abdominal pain.
- Alarm features: weight loss, obstruction, palpable mass, or family history of colorectal malignancy.

Screening Recommendations:

- Screen average-risk adults aged 50–74 every 2 years with FIT (Fecal Immunochemical Test).
- Consider earlier screening (age 40 or 10 years before youngest case) for first-degree relatives with CRC.
- Colonoscopy is diagnostic for positive FIT results or high-risk patients.
- Encourage dietary fiber, reduced red meat, smoking cessation, and physical activity to reduce risk.
- Maintain EMR reminders for overdue screenings and track FIT completion rates.

2. Primary Care Diagnostic Approach:

A systematic approach ensures timely diagnosis and referral.

- History: bleeding pattern, bowel changes, pain, anemia, family history, and weight loss.
- Physical exam: inspect for pallor, perform digital rectal exam for masses or occult bleeding.

Initial investigations:

- FIT or FOBT if not recently done.
- CBC for anemia and iron studies for occult GI bleeding.
- LFTs to screen for liver metastasis if suspected.
- If FIT positive or red-flag symptoms present → urgent colonoscopy (within 2–4 weeks).
- Imaging (CT abdomen/pelvis) may be used if obstruction or advanced disease suspected.
- Avoid empiric iron replacement without completing GI workup.

3. Pre-Referral and Referral Workflow:

Pre-Referral Management:

- Explain the significance of positive FIT or suspicious symptoms to the patient.
- Ensure anemia or bleeding is investigated before labeling as benign cause.
- Correct mild dehydration or anemia prior to referral if safe to do so.
- Document family history and any previous colonoscopy reports.
- Provide reassurance while emphasizing need for timely investigation.

Referral Preparation:

Urgent referral for:

- Positive FIT, rectal bleeding with anemia, or mass on exam.
- Iron-deficiency anemia in men or postmenopausal women.
- Semi-urgent (within 4 weeks) for chronic bowel change without alarm features.
- Attach FIT, CBC, LFT, prior scopes, and medication list (anticoagulants).

- For obstruction or acute bleeding → direct ER referral for CT and surgical consult.
- Confirm receipt of referral and track follow-up completion in EMR.

4. Management, Complications, and Follow-Up

Family doctors play a key role in patient education, supportive care, and survivorship follow-up.

Treatment Overview:

- Surgery – primary treatment for localized disease (segmental resection ± lymph node removal).
- Chemotherapy – adjuvant FOLFOX or CAPOX for stage III or high-risk stage II disease.
- Radiation – for rectal cancer pre- or post-operatively to improve local control.
- Palliative care – for advanced or metastatic disease focusing on quality of life.

Common Complications and Management:

- Post-surgical bowel changes: dietary counseling, stool regulation (fiber, hydration).
- Stoma care: provide education and link to enterostomal therapy nurse.
- Chemotherapy side effects: monitor for neuropathy, cytopenia, mucositis, or diarrhea.
- Fatigue: encourage exercise, screen for anemia or thyroid disease.
- Emotional support: address fear of recurrence and refer to counseling if needed.

Follow-Up Schedule:

• Every 3–6 months for 2 years, then every 6 months to year 5.

• Investigations: CEA every 3–6 months, annual CT chest/abdomen/pelvis for 3 years, and colonoscopy at 1 year post-surgery, then at 3 and 5 years.

• Manage comorbidities, monitor for recurrence, and promote survivorship wellness.

5. Family Doctor's Role – Clinical Scenario (Q&A Format):

CASE: A 56-year-old man presents with a 3-month history of intermittent rectal bleeding, mild fatigue, and a 5 kg weight loss.

Q1. What initial investigations should be ordered?

FIT or FOBT, CBC, ferritin, LFTs, and digital rectal exam. If FIT positive, refer for urgent colonoscopy.

Q2. What findings warrant urgent referral?

Positive FIT, iron-deficiency anemia, or palpable rectal mass.

Q3. What should be discussed with the patient?

Explain possible causes, need for colonoscopy, and early detection improves cure rate.

Q4. What is the GP's role post-diagnosis?**

Coordinate oncology referral, manage symptoms, and provide ongoing psychosocial support.

Q5. How should follow-up be managed after oncology discharge?

Schedule CEA monitoring, ensure surveillance colonoscopies, and encourage healthy lifestyle and adherence to follow-up schedule.

CHAPTER 5:
Endometrial Cancer

1. Recognition and Screening:

Endometrial cancer is the most common gynecologic malignancy in Canada and is often diagnosed early due to postmenopausal bleeding.

- Key symptom: **postmenopausal bleeding** — occurs in >90% of cases.
- Premenopausal red flags: intermenstrual bleeding, prolonged heavy menses, or bleeding after age 45 with risk factors.
- Risk factors: obesity, diabetes, hypertension, nulliparity, unopposed estrogen, polycystic ovary syndrome (PCOS), tamoxifen use, or Lynch syndrome.
- Physical findings: uterine enlargement, cervical stenosis, or adnexal mass (late presentation).
- No population screening; surveillance only for high-risk patients (e.g., Lynch syndrome carriers).
- Document menstrual and reproductive history, medication use, and BMI in EMR.

2. Primary Care Diagnostic Approach:

- Timely evaluation of abnormal uterine bleeding is critical for early detection and improved prognosis.
- History: bleeding pattern, menopausal status, medications (tamoxifen, HRT), family history of gynecologic cancers.
- Physical exam: abdominal and bimanual exam for uterine size/tenderness, and speculum exam for cervical lesions.

Investigations:

- CBC and ferritin for anemia evaluation.
- Transvaginal ultrasound (TVUS): preferred first-line imaging; endometrial thickness >4 mm postmenopause warrants biopsy.
- Endometrial biopsy (office pipelle) for all postmenopausal bleeding or premenopausal abnormal bleeding with risk factors.
- If biopsy not possible in office → refer for hysteroscopy and D&C.
- Avoid empiric progestin therapy before obtaining tissue diagnosis unless advised by specialist.
- Pregnancy test mandatory for reproductive-aged patients before biopsy.

3. Pre-Referral and Referral Workflow:

Pre-Referral Management:

- Explain abnormal findings and need for gynecologic oncology referral.
- Manage anemia and comorbidities (diabetes, hypertension) before surgery or referral.
- Provide reassurance while emphasizing urgency of evaluation; most cases are curable if detected early.
- Avoid hormonal treatment until malignancy excluded.

Referral Preparation:

Urgent referral for:

- Postmenopausal bleeding with thickened endometrium (>4 mm).
- Abnormal biopsy showing hyperplasia with atypia or carcinoma.

- Persistent bleeding despite normal imaging or biopsy (repeat evaluation warranted).
- Semi-urgent referral for abnormal bleeding with risk factors in perimenopausal women.
- Include: TVUS report, biopsy results, CBC, and comorbidity summary in referral letter.
- Coordinate travel and follow-up for rural patients with limited oncology access.

4. Management, Complications, and Follow-Up

Treatment Overview:

- Stage I–II: total hysterectomy with bilateral salpingo-oophorectomy ± lymph node assessment.
- Stage III–IV or high-risk histology: surgery + adjuvant radiation and/or chemotherapy.
- Non-surgical candidates (medically unfit or fertility preservation): progestin therapy (oral or IUD-based).

Primary Care Role:

- Manage anemia, optimize comorbidities, and provide psychological support pre-surgery.
- Postoperatively: monitor wound healing, manage menopausal symptoms, and support rehabilitation.
- Address sexual dysfunction and emotional distress post-treatment.
- Counsel on weight loss, exercise, and diabetes management to reduce recurrence risk.

Follow-Up Schedule:

- Every 3–6 months for first 3 years, every 6–12 months until year 5, then annually.
- Follow-up includes pelvic exam, review of symptoms (bleeding, pain, discharge), and imaging if recurrence suspected.
- Educate patients to report any new vaginal bleeding or pelvic pressure promptly.

5. Family Doctor's Role – Clinical Scenario (Q&A Format):

CASE: A 62-year-old woman presents with postmenopausal bleeding for 2 weeks. She has hypertension, diabetes, and obesity (BMI 34).

Q1. What should be the first diagnostic step?

Order a transvaginal ultrasound to assess endometrial thickness, followed by an office endometrial biopsy if ≥4 mm.

Q2. What findings warrant urgent referral?

Endometrial thickness >4 mm, positive biopsy for atypia/carcinoma, or persistent bleeding with risk factors.

Q3. What supportive measures can be initiated before referral?

Optimize comorbidities (BP, glucose), correct anemia, and provide emotional reassurance.

Q4. What are the GP's responsibilities post-surgery?

Monitor wound healing, manage menopausal symptoms, and ensure adherence to oncology follow-up schedule.

Q5. What long-term follow-up care is needed?

Annual pelvic exams, patient education on recurrence signs, weight management, and mental health support.

CHAPTER 6:
Leukemia

1. Recognition and Screening:

- Leukemia encompasses a group of hematologic malignancies including acute and chronic myeloid and lymphoid leukemias.
- Early symptoms are often nonspecific: fatigue, pallor, bruising, recurrent infections, or unexplained fever.
- Physical findings: pallor, petechiae, hepatosplenomegaly, lymphadenopathy, or bone pain.
- Red flags: sudden severe cytopenias, unexplained weight loss, night sweats, or bleeding diathesis.
- No routine population screening; recognition depends on astute clinical suspicion from blood test abnormalities.
- Family doctors are often the first to detect abnormal CBC patterns (anemia, thrombocytopenia, leukocytosis, or blasts).

2. Primary Care Diagnostic Approach:

- Early detection and rapid coordination with hematology are essential for outcomes, especially in acute leukemias.
- Initial tests: CBC with differential and peripheral smear – key for early recognition.

Findings may include:

- Anemia and thrombocytopenia with or without leukocytosis.
- Presence of blasts or abnormal lymphocytes on smear.

Supportive tests:

- LDH, uric acid, creatinine, calcium, and liver enzymes to assess tumor burden and organ function.
- Coagulation profile if DIC suspected (especially in Acute Promyelocytic Leukemia).
- Flow cytometry and cytogenetic testing performed after hematology referral.
- Chest X-ray if mediastinal mass suspected (T-cell ALL).
- Avoid corticosteroids before confirming diagnosis, as it can obscure morphology and delay classification.

3. Pre-Referral and Referral Workflow:

Pre-Referral Management:

- For suspected acute leukemia, treat as an emergency – arrange same-day hematology contact or ER transfer.
- Ensure IV access, hydration, and baseline labs (CBC, electrolytes, renal and liver function).
- Avoid transfusing platelets or blood before specialist consultation unless hemodynamically unstable.
- Manage fever with empiric broad-spectrum antibiotics after cultures (risk of neutropenia).
- Counsel patient and family about urgency and expected transfer to tertiary care.
- For chronic leukemia (CML/CLL), outpatient referral within 2–4 weeks is appropriate if patient stable.

Referral Preparation:

Urgent referral for:

- Presence of blasts on smear or pancytopenia with symptoms.
- Symptomatic anemia, thrombocytopenia, or infection with abnormal WBC morphology.
- Semi-urgent referral for:

- Asymptomatic lymphocytosis >5 × 10⁹/L or suspected CML with elevated WBC and splenomegaly.
- Include: CBC, smear, electrolytes, uric acid, LDH, renal/liver results, and coagulation profile.
- Document transfusions or antibiotics administered and note any access difficulties (e.g., rural logistics).

4. Management, Complications, and Follow-Up

Treatment Overview:

- Acute Leukemias (AML, ALL): multi-agent chemotherapy ± stem cell transplant.
- Chronic Leukemias (CML, CLL): targeted therapy (tyrosine kinase inhibitors or monoclonal antibodies) and monitoring.
- Palliative care integration for frail or relapsed patients is crucial.

Primary Care Role During Oncology Management:

- Monitor CBC, renal/liver function, and signs of infection or bleeding between oncology visits.
- Manage chemotherapy side effects (nausea, mucositis, fatigue, cytopenias).
- Vaccinations: influenza and pneumococcal (avoid live vaccines).
- Educate on neutropenia precautions (hand hygiene, avoiding raw foods).
- Provide psychological and family support; screen for depression and financial strain.

Common Complications:

- Tumor lysis syndrome – hydration and allopurinol pre-treatment if indicated.
- Infections due to neutropenia – prompt antibiotic initiation.

- Bleeding due to thrombocytopenia – avoid NSAIDs, minimize trauma, and consider transfusion as per hematology.
- Cytopenias post-therapy – monitor closely and coordinate with oncology for supportive transfusions.

Follow-Up After Oncology Discharge:

- Every 3–6 months: CBC, metabolic profile, and review for relapse symptoms.
- Monitor for secondary malignancies and late effects of chemotherapy (cardiac, thyroid, fertility).
- Encourage healthy lifestyle, vaccinations, and smoking cessation.

5. Family Doctor's Role – Clinical Scenario (Q&A Format):

CASE: A 54-year-old man presents with fatigue, easy bruising, and recurrent nosebleeds. His CBC shows Hb 84 g/L, WBC 38 × 10^9/L with 60% blasts, and platelets 28 × 10^9/L.

Q1. What are the immediate next steps?

Confirm smear findings, establish IV access, and arrange same-day transfer to tertiary hematology center.

Q2. What supportive measures should be started?

Hydrate, obtain blood cultures, start empiric antibiotics for fever, and monitor for bleeding.

Q3. What should be avoided before diagnosis confirmation?

Avoid steroids or transfusions unless clinically unstable, as they can interfere with diagnosis and staging.

Q4. How should the family doctor support during treatment?

Provide close outpatient monitoring for infections, cytopenias, and medication adherence. Address emotional and social needs.

Q5. What are key aspects of long-term follow-up?

Monitor for relapse, manage chronic therapy side effects (e.g., imatinib for CML), and coordinate survivorship care.

CHAPTER 7:
Liver Lesion

1. Overview:

Liver lesions are commonly detected incidentally on imaging. Most are benign (hemangioma, cyst, focal nodular hyperplasia), but malignant lesions such as hepatocellular carcinoma (HCC) or metastases must be excluded.

The family physician's role, particularly in rural areas, is to initiate evaluation, interpret reports, and coordinate referral to hepatology or oncology as needed.

2. Risk Factors for Malignancy:

- Chronic viral hepatitis (HBV, HCV)
- Cirrhosis (any cause: alcohol, NAFLD, autoimmune hepatitis)
- Family history of liver cancer
- Aflatoxin exposure or metabolic liver disease (hemochromatosis, alpha-1 antitrypsin deficiency)
- Identifying these factors helps prioritize patients for urgent assessment.

3. Initial Evaluation in Primary Care:

- **History:** Weight loss, jaundice, right upper quadrant pain, pruritus, or prior cancer.
- **Physical Examination:** Hepatomegaly, ascites, spider nevi, jaundice, or cachexia.
- **Laboratory Tests:** CBC, LFTs (ALT, AST, ALP, bilirubin), INR, AFP (alpha-fetoprotein), hepatitis B and C serologies.
- **First-Line Imaging:** Abdominal ultrasound to assess lesion size, number, echogenicity, and vascularity.

4. Imaging and Characterization:

- **Ultrasound:** Initial tool for detection and follow-up.
- **CT or MRI with Contrast:** Used for characterization; arterial enhancement with venous washout suggests HCC.
- **Benign Lesions:** Simple cyst (anechoic, thin wall), hemangioma (peripheral nodular enhancement), focal nodular hyperplasia (central scar).
- **Malignant Lesions:** Irregular margins, arterial hyperenhancement, washout on delayed phase, or multiple lesions.

5. Referral Criteria:

- Lesion >1 cm with suspicious features in a patient with chronic liver disease.
- Elevated AFP >20 µg/L with imaging suspicion.
- New liver lesion in a patient with known malignancy (possible metastasis).
- Indeterminate lesion requiring biopsy or MRI review.
- Referral should be directed to hepatology, gastroenterology, or oncology using provincial pathways.

6. Role After Oncology Discharge:

After treatment for hepatocellular carcinoma or hepatic metastasis, the rural family doctor coordinates ongoing care, including monitoring for recurrence, managing complications, and addressing comorbid liver disease.

Continuity and communication with hepatology and oncology teams are vital.

7. Surveillance and Follow-Up:

- **HCC Surveillance:** Ultrasound every 6 months ± AFP testing.
- **Post-Treatment Imaging:** CT or MRI every 3–6 months during the first 2 years, then annually if stable.
- **Lab Monitoring:** LFTs, AFP, and INR every 3–6 months.
- **Monitor for recurrence symptoms:** jaundice, abdominal pain, weight loss, or ascites.
- The family doctor ensures adherence to surveillance schedules and coordinates results review with specialists.

8. Managing Complications:

- **Cirrhosis-Related:** Ascites (sodium restriction, diuretics), hepatic encephalopathy (lactulose, rifaximin), variceal bleeding prevention (beta-blockers).
- **Post-Resection:** Monitor for infection, bile leak, and nutritional deficits.
- **Post-Ablation or Embolization:** Manage pain, fever, or hepatic decompensation.
- Vaccination against hepatitis A and B is essential if not immune.

9. Health Promotion and Lifestyle:

- Encourage abstinence from alcohol and avoidance of hepatotoxic medications (NSAIDs, acetaminophen >2 g/day).
- Support weight loss and management of diabetes or metabolic syndrome.
- Promote hepatitis B vaccination for household contacts and safe injection practices.
- Counsel regarding balanced diet and physical activity to maintain liver health.

CHAPTER 8:
Lung Cancer

1. Recognition and Screening:

- Lung cancer is a leading cause of cancer death in Canada, but early detection through screening and vigilance for red flags can improve survival.
- Common symptoms: persistent cough, hemoptysis, chest pain, dyspnea, unexplained weight loss, or fatigue.
- Red flags: recurrent pneumonia in the same lobe, voice changes (hoarseness), or new-onset clubbing.
- Paraneoplastic features: SIADH, hypercalcemia, or digital clubbing.

Screening:

- Annual low-dose CT (LDCT) screening for adults aged 55–74 with ≥30 pack-year smoking history who currently smoke or quit within 15 years.
- Discontinue screening after 3 consecutive negative LDCTs or if patient no longer eligible for curative treatment.
- Encourage smoking cessation at every encounter and document smoking history and readiness to quit.
- Use EMR reminders for eligible patients to ensure screening adherence.

2. Primary Care Diagnostic Approach:

Early detection requires vigilance when evaluating respiratory symptoms, especially in smokers or high-risk individuals.

- History: onset and duration of cough, hemoptysis, dyspnea, chest pain, smoking and occupational exposure history.

- Physical exam: signs of clubbing, lymphadenopathy, unilateral wheeze, or consolidation not resolving with antibiotics.

Investigations:

- Chest X-ray: first-line for unexplained cough, hemoptysis, or chest pain lasting >3 weeks.
- Urgent CT chest if abnormal X-ray or high clinical suspicion despite normal film.
- CBC, electrolytes, LFTs, calcium (to assess paraneoplastic or metastatic involvement).
- Sputum cytology may help if endobronchial lesion suspected.
- Avoid empiric antibiotic courses beyond one trial if symptoms persist.
- Consider TB or fungal infection in endemic or high-risk populations before labeling as malignancy.

3. Pre-Referral and Referral Workflow:

Pre-Referral Management:

- Explain the findings to the patient clearly but empathetically, emphasizing need for further imaging/biopsy.
- Manage comorbidities (COPD, CHF) to optimize for diagnostic procedures.
- Manage symptoms such as cough, dyspnea, or pain with appropriate medications (e.g., bronchodilators, analgesics).
- Encourage smoking cessation immediately; provide NRT or pharmacotherapy support.
- Review medications and stop anticoagulants only if biopsy or bronchoscopy planned (after discussion with specialist).
- Ensure oxygen saturation and performance status documented before referral.

Referral Preparation:

• **Urgent referral to oncology/pulmonology for:**

  • Abnormal chest X-ray or CT showing mass, nodule, or lymphadenopathy.
  • Hemoptysis or unexplained weight loss with abnormal imaging.
  • Recurrent or non-resolving pneumonia in the same location.
  • Semi-urgent referral (within 4 weeks): pulmonary nodule <8 mm or indeterminate imaging requiring repeat CT.
  • Attach: imaging reports, lab results, smoking history, comorbidities, and ECOG performance status.
  • Document patient's preferences and social support— important for oncology planning, especially in rural settings.

4. Management, Complications, and Follow-Up:

Family doctors play a critical role in supportive care, management of comorbidities, and long-term survivorship.

Treatment Overview:

  • Early-stage (I-II): surgical resection ± adjuvant chemotherapy or radiotherapy.
  • Locally advanced (III): concurrent chemoradiation ± immunotherapy (durvalumab).
  • Metastatic (IV): systemic therapy (targeted, immunotherapy, or palliative chemotherapy).
  • Palliative care integration from diagnosis improves quality of life and outcomes.

Primary Care Role:

- Manage dyspnea (bronchodilators, oxygen), pain, fatigue, and anxiety.
- Treat infections promptly; educate on warning signs (fever, hemoptysis, worsening breathlessness).
- Address nutritional needs and emotional health; involve social work or home care if needed.
- Monitor for chemotherapy-related toxicities (neutropenia, neuropathy) and immunotherapy side effects (pneumonitis, colitis).

Follow-Up Schedule:

- Post-curative treatment: CT chest every 6 months for 2 years, then annually for 5 years.
- Focus on symptom recurrence, cough, hemoptysis, and weight loss.
- Encourage vaccination (influenza, pneumococcal) and smoking cessation support at each visit.

5. Family Doctor's Role – Clinical Scenario (Q&A Format):

CASE: A 68-year-old man with a 40 pack-year smoking history presents with a 6-week cough and mild hemoptysis. Chest X-ray shows a 3 cm right upper lobe opacity.

Q1. What is the next appropriate step?

Order an urgent CT chest with contrast to evaluate the lesion and refer to a lung cancer rapid diagnostic clinic.

Q2. What should be avoided before diagnosis confirmation?

Avoid starting corticosteroids or antibiotics unless infection is strongly suspected.

Q3. What are key aspects of pre-referral management?

Explain findings empathetically, manage COPD symptoms, and support smoking cessation while expediting referral.

Q4. How should the family doctor support during treatment?

Manage pain, dyspnea, nutrition, and anxiety. Monitor side effects of chemo or immunotherapy and maintain vaccination schedules.

Q5. What is the family doctor's role post-oncology discharge?

Provide surveillance for recurrence, monitor for late toxicities, and coordinate palliative or community support when needed.

CHAPTER 9:
Lymphoma

1. Recognition and Screening:

Lymphoma includes Hodgkin (HL) and Non-Hodgkin (NHL) types, presenting with varied symptoms that often mimic benign conditions.

- Early symptoms: painless lymphadenopathy, night sweats, unexplained weight loss, fever (B-symptoms).
- Other possible findings: fatigue, pruritus, alcohol-induced lymph node pain (HL), or persistent cough/dyspnea from mediastinal mass.
- Red flags: rapidly enlarging lymph node, splenomegaly, or cytopenias on CBC.
- No routine screening in asymptomatic individuals; vigilance in unexplained lymphadenopathy is key.
- Persistent lymph node >2 cm for >4 weeks warrants further evaluation or referral.

2. Primary Care Diagnostic Approach:

A thorough history and physical exam are essential to guide appropriate testing and timely referral.

- **History:** duration and pattern of lymph node enlargement, systemic (B) symptoms, infection history, and autoimmune conditions.
- **Physical exam:** assess all lymph node regions (cervical, axillary, inguinal), liver, and spleen size.

Initial investigations:

- CBC, ESR, LDH, and peripheral smear.
- Liver and renal function tests, calcium, and uric acid (tumor lysis risk).
- Chest X-ray for mediastinal mass or pulmonary involvement.
- HIV, hepatitis B/C testing if risk factors present (can influence subtype and treatment).
- Avoid empiric antibiotics or corticosteroids before biopsy, as these can mask lymphoma morphology.
- Excisional lymph node biopsy is preferred for diagnosis; fine-needle aspiration (FNA) alone is insufficient.
- Document presence/absence of B-symptoms, node size, and location in EMR.

3. Pre-Referral and Referral Workflow:

Pre-Referral Management:

- Counsel patient on need for biopsy and potential diagnosis without inducing alarm.
- Avoid corticosteroids or antibiotics unless infection clearly suspected.
- Address pain, pruritus, or anxiety symptomatically while awaiting referral.
- Check CBC, LDH, and renal/liver function before referral to expedite specialist evaluation.
- Manage symptomatic anemia or thrombocytopenia supportively under hematology guidance.
- For airway compression or spinal cord compression, initiate emergency transfer.

Referral Preparation:

Urgent referral for:

- Rapidly enlarging lymph nodes, B-symptoms, or cytopenias.
- Suspicion of mediastinal or retroperitoneal mass causing compression symptoms.
- Semi-urgent referral (within 2–4 weeks) for isolated, persistent lymphadenopathy without systemic features.
- Include in referral: node size, location, symptom duration, prior imaging, CBC, ESR, LDH, and liver/renal tests.
- Ensure biopsy reports and imaging (if done) are attached for multidisciplinary review.

4. Management, Complications, and Follow-Up

Family physicians play a key role in patient education, supportive management, and survivorship care.

Treatment Overview:

- Hodgkin Lymphoma: ABVD chemotherapy ± radiation for localized disease.
- Non-Hodgkin Lymphoma: treatment depends on histologic subtype and stage (R-CHOP regimen commonly used for diffuse large B-cell lymphoma).
- Indolent lymphomas: often managed with 'watch and wait' under hematology supervision.
- Advanced disease: systemic therapy and palliative interventions as appropriate.

Common Complications:

- Febrile neutropenia – urgent hospital evaluation and IV antibiotics.
- Tumor lysis syndrome – hydration, allopurinol, and monitoring during chemotherapy initiation.

41

- Fatigue and neuropathy – monitor functional status, encourage gentle activity, address nutrition.
- Long-term risks: secondary malignancy, hypothyroidism (post-neck radiation), and cardiac toxicity (anthracyclines).

Follow-Up Schedule:

- During active treatment – monthly or as advised by oncology for toxicity monitoring.
- Post-treatment surveillance: every 3–6 months for 2 years, then annually.
- Focus on recurrence symptoms (new nodes, weight loss, fevers) and psychosocial reintegration.
- Maintain immunizations, bone health, and screening for secondary cancers (breast, thyroid, skin).

5. Family Doctor's Role – Clinical Scenario (Q&A Format)

CASE: A 42-year-old woman presents with a painless neck lump for 6 weeks, intermittent night sweats, and a 4 kg weight loss.

Q1. What should be included in the initial assessment?

History of duration, systemic symptoms, infection exposure, and physical exam of all nodal regions and abdomen for splenomegaly.

Q2. What initial tests should be ordered?

CBC, ESR, LDH, renal/liver profile, chest X-ray, and HIV/HBV/HCV serology if indicated.

Q3. When should referral be made?

Refer urgently if B-symptoms or rapid node growth; semi-urgent if isolated persistent lymphadenopathy >4 weeks.

Q4. How can the family doctor support during oncology treatment?

Monitor for infection, manage chemotherapy side effects, ensure vaccinations, and provide psychosocial support.

Q5. What are key aspects of long-term follow-up?

Surveillance for recurrence, screening for secondary cancers, managing chronic fatigue, and supporting emotional recovery.

CHAPTER 10:
Metastatic Cancer

1. Overview:

Metastatic cancer refers to the spread of malignant cells beyond the primary site, representing advanced disease that is often incurable but manageable.

2. Common Sites of Metastasis and Symptoms**

- **Bone:** Pain (often nocturnal), pathological fractures, hypercalcemia.
- **Liver:** Jaundice, hepatomegaly, right upper quadrant pain, elevated liver enzymes.
- **Lung:** Dyspnea, cough, hemoptysis, pleural effusion.
- **Brain:** Headache, focal neurologic deficits, seizures, cognitive changes.
- **Lymph nodes:** Painless enlargement, compressive symptoms.

The presence of new or unexplained systemic symptoms in a cancer survivor should raise suspicion of metastasis.

3. Initial Assessment in Primary Care:

- **History:** Weight loss, pain pattern, neurologic or respiratory symptoms, prior cancer history.
- **Examination:** Full physical exam focusing on lungs, abdomen, bones, lymph nodes, and neurologic function.
- **Investigations:** CBC, liver and renal panels, calcium, chest X-ray, and targeted imaging (CT/MRI/bone scan) if available.
- Early recognition and communication with oncology can improve symptom control and quality of life.

4. Stabilization in Rural Settings:

- The rural family physician may need to manage acute complications before transfer or consultation:
- **Spinal Cord Compression:** Start dexamethasone 10 mg IV/PO, then 4 mg q6h; arrange urgent MRI and oncology contact.
- **Brain Metastases:** Dexamethasone and anticonvulsants if indicated.
- **Hypercalcemia:** IV fluids and bisphosphonates (zoledronic acid or pamidronate).
- **Pathologic Fractures:** Immobilize, provide analgesia, and refer to orthopedic or oncology specialists.
- Documentation and timely communication with tertiary centers are essential.

5. Symptom Management and Palliative Integration:

- The focus of care shifts to improving quality of life.
- **Pain:** Follow the WHO analgesic ladder (non-opioids → weak opioids → strong opioids). Adjust for renal/hepatic function.
- **Dyspnea:** Low-dose opioids, oxygen if hypoxic, and non-pharmacologic support (fan, positioning).
- **Nausea:** Use metoclopramide, haloperidol, or ondansetron as indicated.
- **Fatigue and Depression:** Address reversible causes and initiate SSRIs or psychostimulants if appropriate.

6. Monitoring and Follow-Up:

- Review every 2–4 weeks or as symptoms change.
- Monitor pain control, medication adherence, and family coping.
- Adjust treatment plans as disease progresses.
- Use telehealth for specialist input and coordinate with hospice programs for seamless care transitions.

7. Support for Caregivers and Families:

- Provide emotional and practical support to caregivers who often face isolation and fatigue in rural communities.
- Educate families about symptom expectations, medication administration, and emergency planning.
- Encourage use of respite care and counseling services when available.

8. End-of-Life Care and Documentation:

- The rural family physician should guide patients and families through end-of-life planning with compassion and cultural sensitivity.
- Document goals of care, DNR orders, and preferred place of death.
- Ensure symptom control, dignity, and spiritual care through collaboration with hospice and palliative programs.
- Post-death support for families should be offered where possible.

CHAPTER 11:
Multiple Myeloma

1. Recognition and Screening:

Multiple Myeloma often presents insidiously and is commonly identified through primary care evaluation for nonspecific symptoms.

- **Early signs:** bone pain (especially back or ribs), fatigue, recurrent infections, or unexplained anemia.
- **Red flags:** hypercalcemia, renal impairment, or pathological fractures.
- **Common mnemonic – CRAB:** Calcium elevation, Renal failure, Anemia, Bone lesions.
- Consider screening for monoclonal gammopathy in patients with persistent anemia or renal dysfunction of unclear cause.
- Family doctors are key to identifying myeloma-related bone pain versus mechanical back pain.
- Routine population screening is not recommended; focus is on early recognition in symptomatic or high-risk patients.

2. Primary Care Diagnostic Approach:

A targeted approach helps differentiate myeloma from other causes of bone pain or cytopenias.

Initial investigations:

CBC, creatinine, calcium, albumin, and total protein.

- Serum protein electrophoresis (SPEP) and immunofixation to detect monoclonal (M) protein.
- Serum free light chain assay (kappa/lambda ratio) – more sensitive for light-chain disease.

- Urine protein electrophoresis (UPEP) or 24-hour urine for Bence-Jones proteins.
- Additional tests (if available): beta-2 microglobulin and LDH as prognostic markers.
- Imaging: skeletal survey or whole-body low-dose CT for bone lesions; MRI for focal pain or compression symptoms.
- Avoid empiric steroid therapy before specialist review unless spinal cord compression suspected.
- Distinguish Multiple Myeloma from MGUS (Monoclonal Gammopathy of Undetermined Significance) and Smoldering Myeloma by M-protein level and end-organ damage.

3. Pre-Referral and Referral Workflow:

Pre-Referral Management:

- Stabilize complications: hydrate if hypercalcemia or renal dysfunction present; avoid nephrotoxic drugs (NSAIDs, contrast).
- Manage pain with acetaminophen or opioids; avoid NSAIDs if renal impairment.
- Correct hypercalcemia with IV fluids and bisphosphonates if available locally.
- Review medications for potential nephrotoxicity or bone marrow suppression.
- Educate the patient on the suspicion of plasma cell disorder and need for urgent hematology review.
- Monitor urine output, renal function, and calcium levels while awaiting referral.

Referral Preparation:

- Urgent hematology/oncology referral for:
- Positive M-protein with CRAB features (anemia, renal failure, bone lesions, hypercalcemia).

- Unexplained cytopenias or renal failure with monoclonal protein.
- Semi-urgent referral for smoldering myeloma without end-organ damage.
- Include all investigations: CBC, SPEP, UPEP, renal profile, calcium, imaging, and symptoms summary.
- Document pain severity, renal function trend, and prior imaging findings.
- Coordinate patient transport and early follow-up for those in rural areas.

4. Management, Complications, and Follow-Up:

Family physicians play an essential role in comorbidity management, toxicity monitoring, and long-term follow-up.

Treatment Overview:

- Combination chemotherapy (bortezomib, lenalidomide, dexamethasone) is standard for induction.
- Autologous stem cell transplant for eligible patients under 70 with good performance status.
- Maintenance therapy (lenalidomide or bortezomib) prolongs remission.
- Bisphosphonates (zoledronic acid) for bone disease prevention and skeletal event reduction.

Primary Care Role in Management:

- Monitor renal function, calcium, hemoglobin, and medication adherence during oncology therapy.
- Provide vaccinations (influenza, pneumococcal, shingles if appropriate).
- Manage infections promptly; avoid live vaccines during immunosuppressive therapy.

- Address neuropathy, fatigue, and anemia; consider erythropoietin if indicated by oncology.
- Screen for and manage mood, anxiety, and social support needs.

Follow-Up Schedule:

- Every 1–3 months during active treatment, then every 3–6 months for remission monitoring.
- Periodic labs: CBC, calcium, creatinine, SPEP, and light chain levels to detect relapse.
- Reinforce bone protection (bisphosphonates, vitamin D, calcium).
- Encourage gentle physical activity and smoking cessation.

5. Family Doctor's Role – Clinical Scenario (Q&A Format):

CASE: A 68-year-old man presents with fatigue, diffuse back pain, and recurrent infections. Blood work shows anemia (Hb 92 g/L), elevated calcium (2.85 mmol/L), and creatinine 180 μmol/L.

Q1. What initial investigations should the family doctor order?

CBC, creatinine, calcium, SPEP, UPEP, and serum free light chain assay to confirm suspicion of myeloma.

Q2. What findings suggest Multiple Myeloma?

Presence of M-protein on electrophoresis, abnormal light chain ratio, anemia, hypercalcemia, renal dysfunction, and lytic bone lesions.

Q3. What should be done before referral?

Hydrate the patient, manage pain, and avoid nephrotoxic medications. Initiate urgent hematology referral.

Q4. What are key complications to monitor in follow-up?

Renal failure, recurrent infections, anemia, bone fractures, and hypercalcemia.

Q5. What is the long-term family doctor role post-oncology care?

Monitor labs for relapse, manage chronic pain, support bone health, address vaccination needs, and coordinate palliative or home-based care if progression occurs.

CHAPTER 12:
Ovarian Cancer

1. Recognition and Screening:

Ovarian cancer often presents late due to vague, nonspecific symptoms. Early recognition of warning signs and timely investigation by family physicians are essential for improving outcomes.

- Common symptoms: abdominal bloating, early satiety, pelvic/abdominal pain, urinary frequency or urgency, unexplained weight loss, or fatigue.
- Red flags: ascites, abdominal mass, or postmenopausal new-onset gastrointestinal symptoms.
- Risk factors: family history of ovarian/breast cancer, BRCA1/2 mutation, Lynch syndrome, nulliparity, endometriosis, and prolonged estrogen exposure.
- Protective factors: oral contraceptive use, breastfeeding, and tubal ligation.

Screening:

- No effective population screening; CA-125 and transvaginal ultrasound are **not recommended** for average-risk women.
- High-risk women (BRCA/Lynch) should be referred to genetic counseling for consideration of risk-reducing salpingo-oophorectomy.
- Encourage annual pelvic exams and documentation of family history of ovarian/breast cancers.

2. Primary Care Diagnostic Approach:

Early evaluation is key in symptomatic women, particularly postmenopausal patients with persistent or unexplained abdominal symptoms.

- **History:** onset, duration, and pattern of bloating, pain, urinary, or GI symptoms; menstrual and family history.
- **Physical exam:** assess for pelvic/abdominal mass, ascites, or lymphadenopathy.

Investigations:

- CBC, electrolytes, LFTs, and renal function (evaluate baseline health).
- CA-125: may be elevated in epithelial ovarian cancer but nonspecific (also elevated in endometriosis, fibroids).
- Transvaginal ultrasound (TVUS): preferred first-line imaging for adnexal masses; note size, complexity, septations, and solid components.
- Pelvic or abdominal CT if TVUS suggests malignancy or ascites present.
- Avoid repeated CA-125 without imaging correlation; this delays diagnosis.
- Document findings and symptom persistence (>12 days/month for 3 months suggests higher suspicion).

3. Pre-Referral and Referral Workflow:

Pre-Referral Management:

- Explain abnormal imaging or lab findings sensitively and discuss next steps.
- Manage pain and bowel symptoms conservatively while awaiting further evaluation.

- Address anxiety and provide emotional support; involve family if appropriate.
- For significant ascites → therapeutic paracentesis and send fluid for cytology (if available).
- Avoid surgical exploration in primary care or general surgery settings without oncology consultation.

Referral Preparation:

Urgent gynecologic oncology referral for:

- Complex adnexal mass on imaging or ascites with elevated CA-125.
- Postmenopausal woman with adnexal mass or CA-125 >35 U/mL.
- Evidence of metastasis (omental caking, pleural effusion).
- Semi-urgent referral for persistent pelvic mass without systemic features.
- Include CA-125, imaging reports, clinical summary, and comorbidities in referral package.
- Coordinate virtual oncology consultation for rural patients if access barriers exist.

4. Management, Complications, and Follow-Up:

Treatment Overview:

- Early-stage (I–II): surgical staging with total hysterectomy, bilateral salpingo-oophorectomy, omentectomy, and lymph node sampling.
- Advanced-stage (III–IV): combination chemotherapy (carboplatin + paclitaxel) ± interval debulking surgery.
- Maintenance therapy (PARP inhibitors) for BRCA-positive advanced disease.
- Palliative care: symptom control for recurrent or metastatic disease.

Primary Care Role:

- Manage chemotherapy side effects: nausea, fatigue, myelosuppression, neuropathy.
- Screen and manage psychological distress, anxiety, or depression.
- Manage comorbidities and coordinate community support (home care, nutrition).
- Encourage physical activity, healthy diet, and smoking cessation.

Follow-Up Schedule:

- Every 3 months for 2 years, every 6 months for 3 years, then annually.
- Follow-up includes pelvic exam, CA-125 (if previously elevated), and symptom review.
- Report recurrence signs promptly: abdominal bloating, early satiety, pelvic pain, or dyspnea (pleural effusion).

5. Family Doctor's Role – Clinical Scenario (Q&A Format):

CASE: A 67-year-old woman presents with progressive abdominal bloating and early satiety for 3 months. On exam, she has shifting dullness and a palpable pelvic mass.

Q1. What are the first investigations?

Order CA-125, transvaginal ultrasound, CBC, LFTs, and electrolytes. If abnormal, proceed with CT abdomen/pelvis.

Q2. What findings indicate malignancy?

Complex adnexal mass, ascites, omental caking, and CA-125 >35 U/mL in postmenopausal woman.

Q3. What should be done before referral?

Relieve symptoms (paracentesis if needed), avoid surgery, manage anxiety, and initiate urgent oncology referral.

Q4. How can the family doctor assist during treatment?

Monitor chemotherapy side effects, provide emotional support, and coordinate multidisciplinary care.

Q5. What follow-up care is needed after treatment?

Pelvic exams and CA-125 monitoring every 3–6 months for 5 years; counsel on recurrence symptoms and provide survivorship care.

CHAPTER 13:
Prostate Cancer –

1. Recognition and Screening:

- Prostate cancer is often asymptomatic in early stages and detected through screening or incidental findings.
- Common symptoms: hesitancy, weak stream, nocturia, urgency, frequency, incomplete emptying, or hematuria.
- Red flags: bone pain, weight loss, anemia, or urinary retention suggesting advanced disease.

Screening:

- Routine PSA screening is *not recommended* for average-risk men under 55 or over 70.
- Shared decision-making for men aged 55–69 regarding PSA testing.
- Digital rectal examination (DRE) may be considered adjunct to PSA in symptomatic patients.
- High-risk groups: African ancestry, strong family history (first-degree relative <65), or BRCA2 mutation — consider earlier screening at 45.
- Document shared decision-making discussions in EMR.

2. Primary Care Diagnostic Approach:

Early evaluation and appropriate testing are essential for timely referral and accurate staging.

- **History:** urinary symptoms, bone pain, erectile dysfunction, hematuria, constitutional symptoms, and family history.
- **Physical exam:** abdominal exam for bladder distension; DRE for prostate size, nodules, or asymmetry.

Investigations:

- PSA (total and free PSA ratio if borderline).
- Urinalysis to exclude infection or hematuria causes.
- CBC, creatinine, and ALP if metastasis suspected.

Imaging (ordered by specialist, but GP should know indications):

- MRI or transrectal ultrasound for local staging.
- Bone scan for PSA >20 ng/mL or symptomatic bone pain.
- Avoid empiric antibiotics unless evidence of prostatitis.
- Repeat PSA after 6–8 weeks if elevated due to transient factors (infection, ejaculation, instrumentation).

3. Pre-Referral and Referral Workflow:

Pre-Referral Management:

- Explain PSA results and the potential implications to the patient.
- Address anxiety and provide balanced information on benefits and harms of biopsy.
- Avoid unnecessary repeat PSA testing before urology referral if elevation persistent.
- Manage concurrent urinary tract infection prior to retesting PSA.
- Review medications (e.g., finasteride lowers PSA by ~50%).
- Provide analgesia and bowel management if obstructive symptoms present.
- Ensure all lab and imaging results are attached to referral.

Referral Preparation:

- Urgent referral: PSA >10 ng/mL, abnormal DRE, hematuria, or systemic symptoms.
- Semi-urgent referral (within 4 weeks): persistent PSA elevation (4–10 ng/mL) after repeat test.
- Routine referral: asymptomatic mild PSA elevation for ongoing monitoring.
- Include PSA trend, family history, medications, and prior imaging in referral letter.
- Document date and method of referral and arrange patient follow-up to confirm urology appointment.

4. Management, Complications, and Follow-Up:

Family doctors play a key role in coordination, symptom control, and survivorship monitoring.

Treatment Overview:

- Active surveillance: for low-risk, localized disease (monitor PSA, DRE, MRI).
- Surgery: radical prostatectomy for localized disease in younger patients.
- Radiation therapy: external beam or brachytherapy for local control.
- Androgen deprivation therapy (ADT): for metastatic or biochemical recurrence.
- Chemotherapy or novel hormonal agents (enzalutamide, abiraterone) for advanced disease.

Complications Managed in Primary Care:

- Urinary incontinence: encourage pelvic floor exercises, refer to physiotherapy.
- Erectile dysfunction: PDE5 inhibitors, vacuum devices, or counseling.
- Hot flashes from ADT: SSRIs, gabapentin, or clonidine as tolerated.
- Osteoporosis prevention in ADT: calcium/vitamin D, DEXA scan, bisphosphonates if indicated.
- Metabolic syndrome on ADT: monitor BP, glucose, and lipids annually.
- Emotional distress: screen for depression and provide mental health support.

Follow-Up Schedule:

- Post-surgery or radiation: PSA every 6–12 months for 5 years, then annually.
- Lifelong surveillance for recurrence or metastasis (bone pain, weight loss, anemia).
- Coordinate care with oncology for hormonal therapy side effects and long-term complications.
- Encourage exercise, weight management, and smoking cessation.

5. Family Doctor's Role – Clinical Scenario (Q&A Format):

CASE: A 64-year-old man presents with nocturia, weak urinary stream, and occasional hematuria. His father was diagnosed with prostate cancer at age 62.

Q1. What are the first steps in evaluation?

Take a full urinary history, perform DRE, and order PSA and urinalysis.

Q2. What results would raise suspicion?

A PSA level above 10 ng/mL or a nodular/asymmetric prostate on DRE requires urgent urology referral.

Q3. How should the family doctor counsel the patient?

Explain that elevated PSA doesn't always mean cancer, discuss potential next steps (biopsy, MRI), and provide reassurance while arranging referral.

Q4. After diagnosis of localized prostate cancer, what is the GP's role?

Coordinate post-surgical or radiation follow-up, manage urinary and sexual complications, and reinforce adherence to specialist care plans.

Q5. How should follow-up be managed after oncology discharge?

Monitor PSA annually, screen for treatment side effects, and support lifestyle changes for cardiovascular and bone health.

CHAPTER 14:
Skin Cancer

1. Recognition and Screening:

- Skin cancer is the most common malignancy in Canada. Early detection significantly improves outcomes, especially for melanoma.
- **Malignant Melanoma:** irregular pigmented lesion with asymmetry, border irregularity, color variation, diameter >6 mm, or evolving appearance (ABCDE criteria).
- **Squamous Cell Carcinoma (SCC):** scaly, crusted, non-healing lesion or firm nodule; may ulcerate or bleed.
- Basal Cell Carcinoma (BCC): pearly papule with telangiectasia, rolled borders, or central ulceration ('rodent ulcer').
- **High-risk features:** rapid growth, pain, bleeding, or recurrence at prior scar site.
- **Risk factors:** fair skin, chronic UV exposure, immunosuppression, prior radiation, and family history of melanoma.
- Encourage patient self-examination and routine full-skin checks for high-risk individuals (e.g., transplant patients).
- No population-wide screening program in Canada; opportunistic clinical skin exams are recommended.

2. Primary Care Diagnostic Approach:

- Accurate clinical evaluation and early biopsy are key for diagnosis and staging.
- History: lesion duration, changes in size/color, bleeding, pain, pruritus, and sun exposure history.
- Physical exam: inspect entire skin surface, assess regional lymph nodes, and document lesion dimensions and features.

Biopsy:

- Excisional biopsy with narrow margins (2 mm) is preferred for suspected melanoma.
- Punch or shave biopsy may be acceptable for large lesions where excision impractical (SCC/BCC).
- Do not perform superficial shave biopsy for suspicious melanomas—can compromise depth assessment.
- Document lesion photos, location, and dermoscopic features if available.
- CBC and imaging only if clinically advanced or nodal/metastatic disease suspected.
- Avoid empiric topical steroids or destructive treatments before biopsy.

3. Pre-Referral and Referral Workflow:

Pre-Referral Management:

- Counsel patient on biopsy results and discuss need for further excision or oncology evaluation.
- Manage wound care and infection prevention post-biopsy.
- Advise strict sun protection and avoidance of tanning beds.
- For high-risk or invasive lesions, assess lymph node status and pain control while awaiting referral.

Referral Preparation:

- Urgent referral to dermatology or surgical oncology for:
- Confirmed invasive melanoma (Breslow depth ≥0.8 mm or ulceration).
- SCC with rapid growth, pain, or perineural invasion on histology.
- Recurrent or aggressive BCC invading deeper tissues.

Semi-urgent referral for:

- Non-healing or suspicious lesions pending definitive excision.
- Include pathology report, lesion photo, biopsy site diagram, and relevant comorbidities in referral letter.
- For rural settings, ensure wound care supplies and patient education provided before travel to specialist.

4. Management, Complications, and Follow-Up:

Treatment Overview:

- **Melanoma:** wide local excision based on Breslow depth ± sentinel lymph node biopsy. Adjuvant immunotherapy for stage III/IV disease (e.g., nivolumab).
- **SCC:** surgical excision with clear margins; radiation for unresectable or advanced lesions.
- **BCC:** surgical excision, curettage, cryotherapy, or topical therapy (imiquimod/5-FU) for superficial lesions.

Primary Care Role:

- Postoperative wound care, scar monitoring, and infection prevention.
- Reinforce sun protection (broad-spectrum sunscreen, clothing, hat).
- Monitor for recurrence or new lesions every 6–12 months for 5 years, lifelong for melanoma.
- Manage treatment side effects: radiation dermatitis, chronic pain, or lymphedema.
- Address psychological effects (disfigurement, anxiety). Offer counseling if needed.

Follow-Up Schedule:

- **Melanoma:** Every 3–6 months for 2 years, every 6–12 months thereafter.
- **SCC/BCC:** Every 6–12 months for first 2 years, then annually.
- Educate patients on self-examination and early reporting of new or changing lesions.

5. Family Doctor's Role – Clinical Scenario (Q&A Format):

CASE: A 59-year-old man presents with a dark irregular mole on his upper back that has increased in size and recently bled. Examination shows an asymmetric lesion, 9 mm in diameter, with irregular borders and multiple shades of brown and black.

Q1. What should be the next step?

Perform an excisional biopsy with 2 mm margins to establish diagnosis and measure Breslow depth.

Q2. What findings require urgent referral?

Pathology confirming invasive melanoma, or any lesion with Breslow depth ≥ 0.8 mm, ulceration, or positive margins.

Q3. What should the family doctor do before referral?

Discuss biopsy results, assess lymph nodes, manage wound care, and provide sun safety counseling.

Q4. How should the family doctor support during treatment?

Coordinate with oncology for staging and immunotherapy; manage pain, wound healing, and mental health.

Q5. What follow-up care is required post-oncology discharge?

Skin exam every 6–12 months, education on self-monitoring, and management of sun protection and emotional wellbeing.

CHAPTER 15:
Thyroid Cancer

1. Recognition and Screening:

- Thyroid cancer often presents as an asymptomatic thyroid nodule detected incidentally. Early recognition and appropriate referral are key to improving outcomes.
- Common presentations: painless thyroid nodule, cervical lymphadenopathy, or incidental imaging finding.
- Red flags: rapid growth, hoarseness, dysphagia, dyspnea, or firm fixed mass.
- High-risk factors: prior neck radiation, family history of thyroid cancer, MEN2 syndrome, or exposure to ionizing radiation.
- Routine population screening is **not recommended**; evaluation is indicated only for clinically detected nodules or risk factors.
- Palpation of thyroid and neck nodes should be part of annual physicals in high-risk patients.

2. Primary Care Diagnostic Approach:

Initial work-up focuses on differentiating benign from malignant nodules using clinical, biochemical, and imaging evaluation.

- **History:** duration, rate of growth, compressive symptoms, voice changes, and radiation exposure.
- **Physical exam:** thyroid size, consistency, tenderness, fixation, and presence of cervical lymphadenopathy.

Investigations:

- Serum TSH: if suppressed, perform radionuclide scan (hot nodules are rarely malignant).
- If TSH normal or high → proceed with ultrasound of thyroid and neck.
- Ultrasound findings suspicious for malignancy: microcalcifications, irregular margins, hypoechogenicity, taller-than-wide shape, or abnormal cervical nodes.
- Fine-needle aspiration (FNA) biopsy recommended for nodules ≥1 cm with suspicious ultrasound features or ≥2 cm if low risk.
- Document nodule size, ultrasound features, and cytology results using the Bethesda system.
- Avoid routine thyroglobulin testing preoperatively—it is not diagnostic.

3. Pre-Referral and Referral Workflow:

Pre-Referral Management:

- Review all lab and imaging results before referral to avoid duplication.
- Manage thyroid dysfunction (hyper/hypothyroidism) as indicated while awaiting surgical review.
- Provide patient education on nodule findings, emphasizing that most thyroid nodules are benign.
- Reassure but emphasize importance of further evaluation if malignancy suspected.
- For compressive symptoms or airway compromise → arrange urgent surgical or emergency ENT referral.

Referral Preparation:

Urgent referral for:

- FNA showing malignancy or suspicious cytology (Bethesda V–VI).
- Rapidly enlarging neck mass or hoarseness with fixed nodule.
- Suspicious cervical lymphadenopathy on ultrasound.
- Semi-urgent referral (within 4 weeks): indeterminate FNA (Bethesda III–IV) or high-risk ultrasound features.
- Attach ultrasound report, cytology results, TSH level, and any prior imaging to referral letter.
- For rural areas, coordinate virtual consults or centralized rapid thyroid assessment programs.

4. Management, Complications, and Follow-Up

Treatment Overview:

- Papillary/Follicular carcinoma: surgical resection (lobectomy or total thyroidectomy) ± radioactive iodine ablation.
- Medullary carcinoma: total thyroidectomy with central neck dissection; evaluate for MEN2 (calcitonin, RET testing).
- Anaplastic carcinoma: urgent oncology/surgical evaluation; palliative focus if unresectable.

Primary Care Role:

- Manage thyroid hormone replacement post-thyroidectomy (levothyroxine to suppress TSH).
- Monitor calcium and vitamin D levels postoperatively (risk of hypocalcemia).
- Provide wound and voice assessment post-surgery; refer to speech therapy for vocal cord paralysis.
- Encourage lifelong adherence to thyroid hormone and follow-up visits.

- Address psychological impact and body image concerns; offer counseling if needed.

Follow-Up Schedule:

- Post-surgery: review at 6–12 weeks, then every 6–12 months with endocrinology.
- Monitoring includes TSH, thyroglobulin (for papillary/follicular types), and neck ultrasound as indicated.
- Screen for recurrence symptoms: neck swelling, dysphonia, dysphagia, or bone pain.
- Encourage smoking cessation and balanced iodine intake.

5. Family Doctor's Role – Clinical Scenario (Q&A Format)

CASE: A 46-year-old woman presents with a slowly enlarging neck lump noticed over 3 months. She has no pain but mild dysphagia. TSH is normal, and ultrasound shows a 1.6 cm hypoechoic thyroid nodule with microcalcifications.

Q1. What is the next appropriate step?

Arrange an ultrasound-guided fine-needle aspiration (FNA) biopsy and review cytology using the Bethesda classification.

Q2. What findings would warrant urgent referral?

FNA results showing Bethesda V–VI (suspicious or malignant) or rapidly enlarging nodule with compressive symptoms.

Q3. What should be done before referral?

Review labs (TSH, calcium), ensure imaging and cytology are complete, and manage any thyroid dysfunction.

Q4. What is the GP's role post-surgery?

Monitor calcium, start levothyroxine, check TSH levels, and ensure wound and voice recovery.

Q5. What are the key points in long-term follow-up?

Annual TSH and thyroglobulin testing, periodic ultrasound, and education on recognizing recurrence signs.

CHAPTER 16:
Thyroid Nodule

1. Initial Evaluation:

- **History:** Prior head/neck radiation, family history of thyroid cancer or MEN-2, rapid growth, dysphagia, hoarseness.
- **Physical Examination:** Assess nodule size, consistency, mobility, lymphadenopathy, and voice changes.
- **Laboratory Tests:** Serum TSH (primary test); if low, perform thyroid scan to assess for hyperfunctioning ("hot") nodules.
- **Ultrasound:** All palpable or incidentally discovered nodules should undergo high-resolution ultrasound to characterize risk.

2. Ultrasound Risk Stratification (TI-RADS/ATA):

Sonographic features suggesting malignancy include:

- Hypoechogenicity
- Irregular margins or extrathyroidal extension
- Microcalcifications
- Taller-than-wide shape
- Increased central vascularity
- Nodules are categorized by risk level to guide biopsy decisions.

3. Indications for Fine-Needle Aspiration (FNA):

- Nodules ≥1 cm with high-risk ultrasound features
- Nodules ≥1.5–2 cm with intermediate risk
- Any size with suspicious lymphadenopathy
- Rapidly enlarging or symptomatic nodules

- In rural areas, ultrasound-guided FNA may be available via regional hospitals; otherwise, refer to endocrinology or surgery.

4. Referral and Communication:

The family physician should refer patients with suspicious cytology (Bethesda III–VI), compressive symptoms, or evidence of local invasion to an endocrinologist or thyroid surgeon.

Use provincial thyroid nodule pathways.

5. Follow-Up and Surveillance:

- **TSH Monitoring:** Maintain TSH suppression as per oncologist recommendation.
- **Thyroglobulin (Tg):** Tumor marker checked every 6–12 months for recurrence.
- **Ultrasound:** Neck ultrasound every 6–12 months initially, then annually if stable.
- **Physical Exam:** Check for cervical nodes and scar changes at each visit.

The family doctor ensures adherence to follow-up schedules and communicates results to the oncology team.

6. Managing Long-Term Complications:

- Hypothyroidism: Lifelong levothyroxine replacement; adjust based on TSH goals.
- Hypocalcemia: Common post-thyroidectomy; monitor calcium and vitamin D levels.
- Voice Changes: Assess for recurrent laryngeal nerve injury; refer to ENT if persistent.
- Fatigue/Weight Gain: Address medication timing and monitor adherence.

- Collaboration with endocrinology is key for dose adjustments.

7. Health Promotion and Survivorship Care:

- Encourage medication adherence, smoking cessation, and balanced diet.
- Educate about radiation safety if recent radioactive iodine therapy.
- Provide psychosocial support, particularly for anxiety related to recurrence.
- Annual preventive care (lipids, bone health, cardiovascular screening) remains important.
- Rural follow-up ensures ongoing patient reassurance and early recognition of recurrence.

PART B:
CLINICAL GUIDE FOR FAMILY PHYSICIANS

CHAPTER 17:
Breaking Bad News in Cancer Care

1. Preparation:

- Choose a quiet, private, and comfortable setting with minimal interruptions.
- Schedule adequate time and ensure the presence of family members or support persons if the patient wishes.
- Review all medical information, diagnostic results, and potential treatment options beforehand.
- Ensure cultural, spiritual, and linguistic needs are respected.
- Mentally prepare yourself for possible emotional responses.

2. The SPIKES Framework:

- **S – Setting up the interview:** Ensure privacy, sit down, make eye contact, and minimize distractions.
- **P – Perception:** Assess the patient's understanding of their condition. Ask, "What have you been told so far?"
- **I – Invitation:** Ask how much information the patient wants: "Would you like me to go through all the details now?"
- **K – Knowledge:** Deliver the news clearly and compassionately. Use simple, non-technical language. Provide information in small chunks and avoid overwhelming details.
- **E – Emotions and Empathy:** Pause to allow emotional reactions. Offer empathetic statements such as, "I can see this is difficult." Silence is therapeutic.
- **S – Strategy and Summary:** Outline the next steps clearly. Discuss treatment options, referrals, and arrange follow-up visits.

3. Communication Tips:

- Use clear, simple, and compassionate language.
- Avoid medical jargon and false reassurance.
- Offer realistic hope and emphasize ongoing support.
- Provide written information and ensure understanding.
- Invite questions and check comprehension regularly.
- Document key discussion points in the medical record.

4. Rural and Remote Considerations:

- Explain referral and follow-up processes clearly when oncology care is distant.
- Utilize tele-oncology services and virtual follow-up when available.
- Provide contact details for provincial cancer agencies and local palliative programs.
- Ensure continuity with the same physician whenever possible.

5. Follow-Up and Support:

- Schedule early follow-up to review the discussion, address questions, and provide emotional support.
- Offer psychosocial, palliative, and community support resources such as the Canadian Cancer Society and Virtual Hospice.
- Encourage ongoing dialogue and reassure patients that care continues despite the diagnosis.

Example Interview: Breaking Bad News – Breast Cancer Stage III

This example illustrates how a family physician can deliver a Stage III breast cancer diagnosis using the SPIKES communication framework. It demonstrates empathy, clarity, and support, with typical patient and family questions and suggested responses.

SETTING THE SCENE

The physician invites Mrs. L (52 years old) and her husband into a private room and ensures they are seated comfortably.

Physician: "Mrs. L, I have the results of your biopsy, and I'd like to discuss them carefully with you. Would you like your husband to be present?"

Patient: "Yes, please."

1. Assessing Perception

Physician: "Before I go into the details, can you tell me what you understand about the tests so far?"

Patient: "I know there was a lump, but I hoped it wasn't cancer."

2. Giving the Diagnosis (Knowledge)

Physician: "The biopsy confirmed that the lump is a breast cancer called invasive ductal carcinoma. It's classified as Stage III, meaning it has spread to nearby lymph nodes but not to other organs. This is serious, but it is treatable."

(Pause. Allow silence for emotions.)

Patient: "Is it curable?"

Physician: "Many women with Stage III breast cancer respond very well to treatment. Our goal is to remove and control the cancer, and in many cases, achieve long-term remission."

3. Responding to Common Questions

Patient: "What caused this? I've been healthy all my life."

Physician: "We rarely know a single cause. Most breast cancers develop from a combination of age, genetics, and hormonal factors. Nothing you did caused this."

Husband: "What are the next steps?"

Physician: "I'll refer you urgently to the provincial breast oncology team. They'll discuss options such as surgery, chemotherapy, and radiation. We'll support you throughout the process."

Patient: "Will I lose my breast or my hair?"

Physician: "Treatment plans vary. Some involve surgery, and some chemotherapy can cause temporary hair loss. We'll make sure you understand each step before starting."

Husband: "Should we tell our children right away?"

Physician: "That's a personal choice. Many families find that honest, age-appropriate conversations help reduce fear. I can connect you with counseling resources if you wish."

4. Closing and Support:

Physician: "I know this is overwhelming. You're not alone. I'll be your main contact as we coordinate with the cancer center. Let's schedule another appointment after you meet the oncology team."

(Provide written information and contact details for support groups and the Canadian Cancer Society helpline.)

CHAPTER 18:
Chemotherapy Side-Effect Management in Rural Hospitals

1. Common Acute Side Effects and Management:

1. Febrile Neutropenia:

- Definition: Temp ≥38°C, ANC <0.5 × 10⁹/L.
- Action: Give broad-spectrum IV antibiotics within 60 minutes.
- Example: Piperacillin-tazobactam 4.5 g IV q6h or meropenem 1 g IV q8h.
- Obtain CBC, blood cultures ×2, lactate, renal function.

2. Nausea and Vomiting:

- Ondansetron 8 mg IV/PO q8h ± dexamethasone 4 mg IV/PO q12h.
- Add metoclopramide or olanzapine if refractory.

3. Mucositis:

- Encourage saline rinses, "magic mouthwash," hydration, soft foods.
- Avoid alcohol-based mouthwash or acidic foods.

4. Diarrhea (especially irinotecan):

- Loperamide 4 mg PO, then 2 mg q2h until symptom-free ×12 h.
- Rule out C. difficile and dehydration; replace fluids/electrolytes.

5. Extravasation Injury:

- Stop infusion immediately, aspirate drug (do not flush line).
- Apply cold compress except for vinca alkaloids (use warm).
- Consult oncology for antidotes (e.g., hyaluronidase, dexrazoxane).

6. Dehydration / Acute Kidney Injury:

- IV fluids (0.9% NaCl), monitor renal function and urine output.
- Avoid NSAIDs and nephrotoxic drugs.

7. Anemia or Thrombocytopenia:

- Transfuse RBCs if Hb <80 g/L or symptomatic.
- Platelet transfusion if <10 × 10^9/L or bleeding.

8. Allergic Reactions (Taxanes, Monoclonals):

- Stop infusion, give **Epinephrine 0.3–0.5 mg IM (1:1000)**.
- Oxygen, IV fluids, diphenhydramine 50 mg IV, hydrocortisone 100 mg IV.
- Monitor airway and prepare for transfer if severe.

References:

- BC Cancer. *Systemic Therapy Emergency Management Guidelines.*
- Alberta Health Services. *Rural Cancer Treatment Complication Pathway.*
- Cancer Care Ontario. *Chemotherapy Toxicity Management Tools.*
- Canadian Cancer Society. *Managing Side Effects of Cancer Treatment.*

- CMAJ. *Approach to Chemotherapy Complications in Non-Tertiary Settings (Open Access).*

CHAPTER 19:
Common Oncology Drug Interactions & Contraindications

1. Common High-Risk Drug Interactions:

1 Warfarin + Chemotherapy (5-FU, Capecitabine, Tamoxifen): ↑ INR — monitor frequently or use LMWH instead.

2 CYP3A4 Inhibitors (macrolides, azoles, grapefruit) + TKIs (imatinib, erlotinib): ↑ serum levels and toxicity.

3 Dexamethasone + Diabetes/Hypertension Medications: Worsens glycemic and blood pressure control.

4 SSRIs (fluoxetine, paroxetine) + Tamoxifen: CYP2D6 inhibition ↓ tamoxifen activity — prefer sertraline or citalopram.

5 Antiepileptics (phenytoin, carbamazepine) + Chemotherapy: ↓ chemotherapy efficacy and ↑ toxicity.

6 Allopurinol + 6-Mercaptopurine / Azathioprine: ↑ marrow toxicity — avoid combination or reduce dose.

7 Methotrexate + NSAIDs or TMP-SMX: ↑ renal and marrow toxicity — avoid or monitor renal function and CBC.

8 ACE inhibitors / ARBs + Cisplatin: ↑ renal dysfunction — monitor creatinine closely.

9 QT-Prolonging Drugs (ondansetron, fluoroquinolones) + Anthracyclines / TKIs: ↑ arrhythmia risk — ECG monitoring required.

RURAL ONCOLOGY POCKET GUIDE

2. Common Contraindications:

- **Pregnancy:** Methotrexate, lenalidomide, thalidomide, tamoxifen (teratogenic).
- **Severe Hepatic Impairment:** Avoid vinca alkaloids and doxorubicin.
- **Severe Renal Impairment:** Avoid cisplatin; adjust methotrexate and capecitabine doses.
- **Cardiac Failure:** Avoid anthracyclines and trastuzumab.
- **Severe Infection or Neutropenia:** Delay cytotoxic therapy until recovery.

References:

- BC Cancer. Drug Interaction Database & Systemic Therapy Guidelines.
- Alberta Health Services. Oncology Drug Safety and Monitoring Pathway.
- Cancer Care Ontario. Drug Interaction Management Tables.
- Canadian Cancer Society. Managing Medicines Safely During Cancer Treatment.

CHAPTER 20:
Medical Assistance in Dying (MAID)

1. Eligibility Criteria

A person must:

- Be at least 18 years old and capable of making health decisions.
- Be eligible for publicly funded health services in Canada.

Have a grievous and irremediable medical condition, defined as:

- Serious and incurable illness, disease, or disability.
- Advanced state of irreversible decline in capability.
- Enduring suffering that is intolerable and cannot be relieved under conditions acceptable to the patient.
- Make a voluntary request not due to external pressure.
- Provide informed consent after being fully informed of palliative and other options.

2. Safeguards and Assessment Process:

- Two independent MAID assessors must confirm eligibility.
- Written request signed before one independent witness.

Reflection period:

- Waived if death is reasonably foreseeable.
- 90 days minimum if death is not reasonably foreseeable.
- The person must be capable of providing consent immediately before MAID is provided (unless prior waiver of final consent was arranged under specific circumstances).
- Physicians or nurse practitioners may provide or administer MAID directly or via prescription for self-administration.

3. Role of the Family Physician in Rural Practice:

- Provide balanced information about MAID, palliative care, and psychosocial supports.
- Conduct or participate in eligibility assessments where qualified.
- Refer patients to provincial MAID coordination services (available 24/7 in all provinces).
- Ensure timely access to symptom management and family counseling.
- Respect conscientious objection, but ensure **effective referral** to another provider or MAID coordination team.

4. Ethical and Cultural Considerations:

- Uphold dignity, compassion, and autonomy while respecting diversity of beliefs.
- Engage in shared decision-making with patients and families.
- Incorporate cultural, spiritual, and religious perspectives, particularly in Indigenous and faith-based communities.
- Document all discussions carefully, including alternative care options offered.

References open access

1. Health Canada. Medical Assistance in Dying (MAID) – Guidance for Health Professionals. https://www.canada.ca/en/health-canada/services/medical-assistance-dying.html

2. Canadian Medical Association (CMA). Policy on MAID and Physician Roles. https://www.cma.ca

3. Canadian Virtual Hospice. MAID Information and Support. https://www.virtualhospice.ca

4. Provincial MAID Coordination Services: Saskatchewan, Alberta, BC, Ontario – publicly listed contact portals.

5. Canadian Cancer Society. End-of-Life Options and Supportive Care. https://cancer.ca/en

CHAPTER 21:
Oncologic Emergencies

1. Neutropenic Sepsis

1. Recognition in Rural/ER Settings:

- Occurs in patients on chemotherapy with absolute neutrophil count (ANC) <0.5 × 10^9/L or expected to fall below this within 48 hours.
- May present with fever >38°C, chills, hypotension, tachycardia, or vague symptoms. Fever may be absent in severely immunosuppressed patients.
- Always treat as life-threatening.

2. Immediate Management in Rural Setting:

- Obtain vitals, oxygen, IV access, and start fluids.
- Draw CBC, blood cultures (x2 sites), urinalysis, CXR if respiratory symptoms.
- Start empiric IV broad-spectrum antibiotics within 60 minutes:
- Piperacillin-tazobactam 4.5 g IV q6h OR Cefepime 2 g IV q8h.
- Add **vancomycin** if hemodynamically unstable or skin/line infection suspected.
- Avoid rectal exams or IM injections.
- If febrile and hypotensive: start sepsis protocol (fluids, vasopressors if needed).

3. Referral and Transfer:

- If unstable, arrange urgent transfer to tertiary or regional cancer centre after initial stabilization.
- Continue IV antibiotics during transfer and monitor vitals closely.

4. Post-Stabilization Monitoring:

- Daily CBC, renal function, cultures, and antibiotic reassessment.
- Avoid NSAIDs; monitor for mucositis, diarrhea, and line infection.

2. Spinal Cord Compression

1. Recognition in Rural/ER Settings:

- Suspect in any cancer patient with new back pain, weakness, sensory changes, or urinary retention.
- Common primaries: breast, prostate, lung, myeloma, lymphoma.
- Pain often precedes neurologic deficits by days to weeks.

2. Immediate Management in Rural Setting:

- Do not delay steroids: Dexamethasone 10 mg IV bolus, then 4 mg IV q6h.
- Strict bed rest and spinal precautions.
- Urgent MRI of the entire spine (if available) or CT if MRI not possible.
- Manage pain with opioids; avoid NSAIDs if renal risk.

3. Referral and Transfer:

- Urgent transfer to tertiary centre with neurosurgery or radiation oncology.
- Continue IV dexamethasone during transfer.
- Notify oncology for consideration of radiation or surgical decompression.

4. Post-Stabilization Monitoring:

- Document neurologic exam q4h.
- Bladder care and prevent pressure sores.

- Supportive physiotherapy post-treatment.

3. Superior Vena Cava (SVC) Syndrome:

1. Recognition in Rural/ER Settings:

- Caused by obstruction of the SVC from tumor (commonly lung cancer, lymphoma) or thrombosis.
- Symptoms: facial/neck swelling, dyspnea, distended neck/chest veins, cough, headache, or syncope.

2. Immediate Management in Rural Setting:

- Elevate head of bed, provide oxygen.
- Avoid upper extremity IV lines if possible.
- Dexamethasone 8 mg IV q8h (reduces edema in malignant cases).
- If significant respiratory distress, consider gentle diuretics.
- Anticoagulation if catheter-related thrombosis suspected.

3. Referral and Transfer:

- Urgent oncology consultation.
- Transfer to tertiary centre for CT chest with contrast, tissue diagnosis, and possible stenting or radiation.
- Continue supportive care and dexamethasone during transfer.

4. Post-Stabilization Monitoring:

- Monitor airway and oxygen saturation continuously.
- Reassess for signs of cerebral edema or airway obstruction.
- Manage anxiety and dyspnea supportively.

4. Hypercalcemia of Malignancy:

1. Recognition in Rural/ER Settings:

- Common in breast, lung, and myeloma patients.
- Symptoms: confusion, weakness, nausea, vomiting, constipation, polyuria, dehydration, and arrhythmias.
- Defined as calcium >2.6 mmol/L (corrected for albumin).

2. Immediate Management in Rural Setting:

- **Rehydrate aggressively:** Normal saline IV 200–300 mL/hr (adjust for cardiac status).
- **Loop diuretics:** Furosemide 20–40 mg IV q12h only after rehydration.
- **Bisphosphonate:** Zoledronic acid 4 mg IV over 15 min (if available) OR Pamidronate 60–90 mg IV over 2–4 hrs.
- **Calcitonin:** 4 IU/kg SC/IM q12h for rapid calcium reduction if symptomatic.
- Stop calcium/vitamin D supplements.

3. Referral and Transfer:

- Admit if calcium >3.5 mmol/L or symptomatic.
- Refer to oncology for further management and evaluation of underlying malignancy.
- Arrange follow-up for repeat calcium and renal function in 24–48 hrs.

4. Post-Stabilization Monitoring:

- Monitor calcium, creatinine, and urine output q12–24h.
- Treat nausea, delirium, and dehydration.
- Encourage oral fluids if able; prevent recurrence via malignancy control.

5. Tumor Lysis Syndrome:

1. Recognition in Rural/ER Settings:

- Occurs when rapid tumor cell breakdown releases intracellular contents, leading to hyperkalemia, hyperphosphatemia, hypocalcemia, and hyperuricemia.
- Common in high-grade lymphomas, leukemias, or bulky tumors after chemotherapy or spontaneously.
- Symptoms: weakness, nausea, muscle cramps, arrhythmia, oliguria, or seizures.

2. Immediate Management in Rural Setting:

- Begin aggressive IV hydration: Normal saline 200–300 mL/hr (adjust for cardiac status).
- Stop all potassium- or calcium-containing fluids.
- Allopurinol 300 mg PO daily (if uric acid not yet elevated) or **Rasburicase 0.2 mg/kg IV (if available) if uric acid >475 µmol/L.
- Monitor ECG and correct hyperkalemia urgently if present.
- Monitor urine output; consider loop diuretics if oliguric.

3. Referral and Transfer:

- Urgent oncology/nephrology consult.
- Transfer to tertiary hospital if creatinine rising, K^+ >6 mmol/L, or arrhythmias develop.
- Continue hydration and ECG monitoring during transfer.

4. Post-Stabilization Monitoring:

- Monitor K^+, Ca^{2+}, phosphate, uric acid, and creatinine q6–12h.
- Maintain urine output >100 mL/hr.
- Avoid nephrotoxins (NSAIDs, contrast).

6. Malignant Pericardial Effusion / Cardiac Tamponade

1. Recognition in Rural/ER Settings:

- Occurs in advanced lung, breast, or lymphoma cancers.
- Symptoms: dyspnea, orthopnea, chest pain, tachycardia, hypotension, distended neck veins, muffled heart sounds.
- ECG: low voltage QRS or electrical alternans.
- Treat as an emergency if tamponade suspected.

2. Immediate Management in Rural Setting:

- Elevate head of bed, give oxygen.
- IV fluids to maintain preload (NS bolus 500–1000 mL).
- Avoid diuretics or vasodilators.
- If tamponade evident (shock, pulsus paradoxus): prepare for urgent pericardiocentesis if trained and equipped.
- Send pericardial fluid for cytology and culture if drainage performed.

3. Referral and Transfer:

- Immediate transfer to tertiary centre (cardiology/thoracic surgery).
- Continue IV fluids and monitor vitals continuously.
- Coordinate with oncology for further management (pericardial window or percutaneous drainage).

4. Post-Stabilization Monitoring:

- Monitor ECG, BP, and urine output.
- Evaluate for recurrence and adjust cancer therapy accordingly.
- Address anxiety and dyspnea supportively.

7. Increased Intracranial Pressure / Brain Metastases

1. Recognition in Rural/ER Settings:

- Brain metastases are common in lung, breast, and melanoma.
- Symptoms: headache (worse in morning), vomiting, vision changes, focal deficits, or seizures.
- Late signs: altered consciousness, papilledema, or Cushing triad (bradycardia, hypertension, irregular respiration).

2. Immediate Management in Rural Setting:

- Elevate head of bed 30, maintain airway and oxygenation.
- Dexamethasone 10 mg IV bolus, then 4 mg IV q6h to reduce edema.
- Mannitol 0.25–1 g/kg IV over 20 min if severe symptoms or signs of herniation.
- Treat seizures with levetiracetam 1 g IV; avoid lumbar puncture.
- Maintain BP and avoid hypoxia or hypotension.
- 3. Referral and Transfer:
- Urgent transfer to tertiary centre with neurosurgery or radiation oncology.
- Continue dexamethasone and oxygen during transfer.
- CT head (if available) before transfer to rule out hemorrhage.

8. Pathologic Fractures / Bone Metastases

1. Recognition in Rural/ER Settings:

- Bone metastases are common in breast, prostate, lung, and thyroid cancers.
- Symptoms: localized pain, swelling, deformity, or inability to bear weight.

- Fracture may occur after minimal trauma.
- Common sites: spine, pelvis, femur, and humerus.

2. Immediate Management in Rural Setting:

- Immobilize affected limb or spine.
- Provide analgesia (opioids ± acetaminophen).
- Obtain X-rays or CT of the affected area.
- Manage hypercalcemia if present (hydration, bisphosphonate).
- Begin DVT prophylaxis if immobilized.

3. Referral and Transfer:

- Transfer to orthopedic or oncology centre for fixation, radiation, or systemic therapy.
- If spinal instability or neurologic symptoms: urgent transfer to neurosurgery.
- Communicate imaging and labs prior to transfer.

4. Post-Stabilization Monitoring:

- Pain management, physiotherapy, and fall prevention.
- Continue bone-strengthening agents (zoledronic acid or denosumab).
- Address emotional and palliative needs for advanced disease.

CHAPTER 22:
Opioid Options

1. Common Opioid Options and Typical Doses (Adults, Opioid-Naïve)

- **Morphine:** 2.5–5 mg PO q4h or 1–2 mg SC q4h (titrate).
- Hydromorphone:** 0.5–1 mg PO q4h or 0.25–0.5 mg SC q4h.
- **Oxycodone:** 2.5–5 mg PO q4–6h.
- **Fentanyl (Transdermal):** Start at 12–25 mcg/hr patch (only for opioid-tolerant).
- **Methadone:** See below (specialist guidance required).
- Breakthrough dose 10% of total 24-hour opioid dose, q1h PRN (PO or SC).
- Equianalgesic Oral Doses (approximate):
- Morphine 10 mg = Hydromorphone 2 mg = Oxycodone 5 mg.
- Morphine 10 mg PO = Morphine 5 mg SC = Hydromorphone 1 mg SC.

2. Methadone – Indications and Dosing:

- Methadone is effective for neuropathic or refractory pain, particularly when other opioids cause adverse effects or tolerance.
- **Starting dose:** 1–2.5 mg PO q8h (opioid-naïve); 75–90% dose reduction when rotating from other opioids.
- **Titration:** Increase every 5–7 days under expert supervision (nonlinear conversion).
- **Cautions:** Prolonged QTc (>450 ms), drug interactions (CYP3A4), and accumulation risk.

- Specialist consultation strongly recommended before initiating or converting.
- **Advantages:** No active metabolites, safe in renal impairment, long half-life.
- **Adjuvants:** Combine with acetaminophen, NSAIDs, or corticosteroids for multimodal control.

3. Opioid Conversion and Rotation (Approximate Ratios):

Used when switching opioids due to side effects or poor control.

1. Calculate total 24-hour opioid dose.

2. Convert to morphine equivalent using converstion table

3. Reduce by 25–50% for incomplete cross-tolerance.

Example: Patient on 60 mg oral morphine/24h → switch to hydromorphone PO = 12 mg/day (divide q4h).

4. Recognition and Management of Common Side Effects:

- **Constipation:** Prevent with senna 2 tabs PO BID ± lactulose 15–30 mL PO daily.
- **Nausea:** Haloperidol 0.5–1 mg PO/SC q8h or metoclopramide 10 mg PO/SC q6h.
- **Sedation:** Usually transient; reduce dose or rotate opioid if persistent.
- **Delirium:** Haloperidol 0.5–1 mg PO/SC q4h; investigate reversible causes.
- **Respiratory Depression:** Stop opioid, give oxygen, and if severe: Naloxone 0.04 mg IV q2–3 min to effect (avoid full reversal in chronic users).

CHAPTER 23:
Palliative & Supportive Care for Rural and Family Physicians

1. Pain Management:

1. Recognition and Assessment:

Assess pain using a 0–10 scale. Classify as nociceptive (somatic/visceral) or neuropathic. Evaluate site, pattern, and breakthrough pain.

2. Non-Pharmacologic Measures:

- Positioning, massage, heat/cold application.
- Relaxation, guided imagery, spiritual and psychosocial support.
- Occupational and physical therapy for mobility.

3. Pharmacologic Management (WHO Analgesic Ladder):

- **Step 1:** Mild pain – Acetaminophen 500–1000 mg PO q6h; ± NSAID (ibuprofen 400 mg PO q8h).
- **Step 2:** Moderate pain – Add opioid: Morphine 2.5–5 mg PO q4h or Hydromorphone 0.5–1 mg PO q4h.
- **Step 3:** Severe pain – Morphine 5–10 mg PO q4h or 2 mg SC q4h; titrate.
- Breakthrough: 10% of total 24-hour dose PRN q1h.
- Neuropathic pain: Gabapentin 100–300 mg PO HS, titrate to 900–1800 mg/day.
- Adjuvants: Dexamethasone 4 mg PO daily for bone pain.

2. Nausea and Vomiting:

1. Recognition and Assessment:

Common in advanced cancer from medications, metabolic issues, bowel obstruction, or CNS metastases. Determine etiology (e.g., opioid, uremia, increased ICP).

2. Non-Pharmacologic Measures:

- Small, frequent meals and clear fluids.
- Elevate head of bed, maintain hydration.
- Avoid strong odors; provide calm environment.

3. Pharmacologic Management:

- Haloperidol 0.5–1 mg PO/SC q8h** (dopamine blockade).
- Metoclopramide 10 mg PO/SC q6h** (prokinetic).
- Ondansetron 4–8 mg PO/IV q8h** (serotonin blockade).
- Dexamethasone 4 mg PO/IV q12h** for increased ICP or liver metastases.
- Rotate agents based on cause and response.

3. Dyspnea:

1. Recognition and Assessment:

Dyspnea is subjective breathlessness common in lung cancer, CHF, COPD, or metastases. Assess anxiety, oxygen saturation, and signs of fluid overload.

2. Non-Pharmacologic Measures:

- Position upright; use a fan toward the face.
- Relaxation techniques, reassurance.
- Oxygen only if hypoxemic (SpO_2 <90%).

3. Pharmacologic Management:

- Morphine 2.5 mg PO or 1 mg SC q1h PRN, titrate for comfort.
- Lorazepam 0.5–1 mg SL q4h PRN for anxiety-related dyspnea.
- Dexamethasone 4 mg PO daily for airway edema or lung metastases.
- Nebulized saline or bronchodilators if obstructive component.
- Furosemide if due to pulmonary edema.

4. Constipation:

1. Recognition and Assessment:

Common due to opioids, dehydration, reduced mobility, or tumor compression. Assess stool frequency, consistency, and contributing medications.

2. Non-Pharmacologic Measures:

- Encourage fluids and fiber if feasible.
- Mobility as tolerated.
- Abdominal massage, toileting routine.

3. Pharmacologic Management:

- **Stimulant laxative:** Senna 8.6 mg 2 tabs PO BID ± Docusate 100 mg PO BID.
- **Osmotic:** Lactulose 15–30 mL PO daily or PEG 17 g in water daily.
- **Refractory cases:** Bisacodyl 10 mg suppository daily or SC Methylnaltrexone 8–12 mg q48h for opioid-induced constipation.

5. Delirium (Terminal Agitation / Confusion):

1. Recognition and Assessment:

Delirium is acute confusion with fluctuating consciousness, agitation, or hallucinations. Causes: infection, dehydration, metabolic issues, opioids, or brain metastases.

2. Non-Pharmacologic Measures:

- Reorient patient frequently; provide familiar faces.
- Reduce noise, ensure lighting and safety.
- Address reversible causes (infection, retention, constipation).

3. Pharmacologic Management:

- Haloperidol 0.5–1 mg PO/SC q4h PRN, titrate up to 5 mg/24h.
- Methotrimeprazine 6.25–12.5 mg SC q8h PRN for agitation or restlessness.
- Midazolam 1–2 mg SC q1h PRN for severe terminal agitation.
- Avoid benzodiazepines unless for palliative sedation or alcohol withdrawal.

CHAPTER 24:
Role of the Family Doctor in Rural Emergency Settings: When to Call an Oncologist

1. Situations Requiring Immediate Oncology Consultation:

1. New or Suspected Oncologic Emergency:

- Spinal cord compression (back pain, weakness, sensory loss).
- Superior vena cava syndrome (facial swelling, dyspnea, venous distention).
- Tumor lysis syndrome (AKI, hyperkalemia, hyperuricemia).
- Neutropenic sepsis (fever $\geq$38°C, ANC <0.5×10^9/L).
- Hypercalcemia of malignancy with altered mental status or arrhythmia.

2. Severe Treatment Complications:

- Cytopenias or febrile neutropenia after chemotherapy.
- Bleeding due to thrombocytopenia or DIC.
- Mucositis, dehydration, or intractable nausea/vomiting.
- Acute kidney injury after contrast or nephrotoxic drugs.

3 Suspected Recurrence or New Metastasis:

- New focal pain, neurological deficits, or mass.
- Rapidly enlarging lymph node or unexplained organ dysfunction.

4. End-of-Life and Palliative Transitions:

- Uncontrolled pain or dyspnea despite escalation.
- Clarification of prognosis or goals of care.
- MAID eligibility, hospice coordination, or transport decisions.

5. Practical Steps for Rural Settings:

- Stabilize patient first (airway, breathing, circulation, analgesia, fluids, antibiotics).
- Obtain essential labs/imaging before calling (CBC, electrolytes, calcium, renal panel).
- Document ECOG performance status and recent treatment history.
- Use provincial oncology on-call lines or tele-oncology consultation.

CHAPTER 25:
Tumor Markers – Comprehensive Clinical Guide for Family Physicians

1. Overview:

Tumor markers are biological substances—usually proteins— produced by cancer cells or by the body in response to malignancy. They can aid in diagnosis, prognosis, treatment monitoring, and detecting recurrence, but rarely confirm cancer alone.

- **Main roles:** diagnosis support, staging, prognosis, treatment response, recurrence monitoring.
- **Limitations:** not disease-specific, may be elevated in benign conditions, and poor screening tools for asymptomatic patients.
- Family doctors should use tumor markers only after clinical evaluation and never as first-line screening in healthy individuals.

2. When to Order Tumor Markers:

When indicated:

- To support diagnosis when malignancy is clinically or radiologically suspected.
- To monitor known malignancy after treatment or during remission follow-up (per oncology plan).
- To assess prognosis or recurrence risk in coordination with oncology specialists.

When not indicated:

- Routine screening of asymptomatic patients (e.g., CA-125, CEA).
- Unexplained elevations without clinical correlation should not trigger extensive testing without consultation.
- Always interpret tumor markers alongside history, exam, and imaging findings.

3. Common Tumor Markers and Clinical Context:

PSA (Prostate-Specific Antigen):

- Elevated in prostate cancer, BPH, prostatitis, or after catheterization/intercourse.
- Screening recommended for men aged 50–70 (40–50 if high-risk) after shared decision-making.
- If >4.0 ng/mL or rising trend → repeat after 6–8 weeks and refer if persistently elevated.

CA-125:

- Marker for epithelial ovarian and endometrial cancers.
- Elevated in benign conditions (fibroids, endometriosis, liver disease).
- Use only for evaluation of pelvic mass or monitoring known ovarian cancer.

CEA (Carcinoembryonic Antigen):

- Used for colorectal, gastric, pancreatic, lung, and breast cancers.
- Elevated in smokers and liver disease; not for screening.
- Used mainly for follow-up post colorectal cancer resection.

AFP (Alpha-Fetoprotein):

- Elevated in hepatocellular carcinoma and germ cell tumors (testicular, ovarian).
- Order in chronic hepatitis or cirrhosis patients with rising levels and abnormal imaging.

β-hCG (Beta-Human Chorionic Gonadotropin):

- Marker for germ cell tumors and trophoblastic disease.
- May be elevated in testicular tumors or certain ovarian cancers.

CA 19-9:

- Marker for pancreatic, biliary, and gastric cancers.
- May rise in cholestasis, gallstones, or pancreatitis.
- Order only when imaging suggests pancreatic pathology.

LDH (Lactate Dehydrogenase):

- Non-specific marker; reflects tumor burden in lymphoma, leukemia, or germ cell tumors.
- Useful for prognosis and relapse monitoring.

Thyroglobulin:

- Marker for differentiated thyroid carcinoma recurrence post-thyroidectomy.
- Always interpret with anti-thyroglobulin antibody levels.

Calcitonin:

- Marker for medullary thyroid carcinoma.
- Order in patients with thyroid nodules and family history of MEN2 syndrome.

CA 15-3 / CA 27.29:

- Used for monitoring breast cancer recurrence, not screening.
- May rise in benign breast or liver diseases.

4. Next Steps After Abnormal Results:

- Confirm results by repeating the test after 4–6 weeks if no clinical correlation.
- Review history and perform full clinical exam for cancer-related symptoms.
- Order directed imaging (e.g., ultrasound, CT, or MRI) based on suspected primary site.
- Discuss abnormal or unexplained results with oncology or internal medicine before further testing.
- Avoid serial testing without specialist input—may lead to unnecessary anxiety and costs.
- In patients with known malignancy, use same lab and assay for serial monitoring to ensure consistency.

5. Family Doctor's Role in Monitoring and Follow-Up:

- Integrate tumor markers into comprehensive follow-up plans established by oncology.
- Reinforce importance of attending oncology appointments and imaging follow-ups.
- Manage anxiety and expectations—educate that mild fluctuations may not indicate recurrence.
- Track trends rather than single values (rising, stable, or falling).
- Document results clearly in EMR and communicate results promptly to patients and oncology teams.
- In rural settings, coordinate local lab draws and virtual oncology consultations.

Unified Reference

1. Canadian Partnership Against Cancer (CPAC). National Cancer Control and Person-Centred Survivorship Framework. https://www.partnershipagainstcancer.ca

2. Canadian Cancer Society. Cancer Information, Screening, Diagnosis, and Follow-Up Resources. https://cancer.ca/en

3. Canadian Task Force on Preventive Health Care (CTFPHC). Screening Guidelines for Major Cancers. https://canadiantaskforce.ca

4. Cancer Care Ontario (CCO). Clinical Pathways and Symptom Management Guidelines. https://www.cancercareontario.ca

5. BC Cancer Agency. Provincial Cancer Management Guidelines and Screening Programs. https://www.bccancer.bc.ca

6. Alberta Health Services (AHS). Cancer Care Clinical Practice Guidelines. https://www.albertahealthservices.ca/info/cancerguidelines.aspx

7. Canadian Urological Association (CUA). Prostate Cancer Guidelines (2023). https://www.cua.org

www.ingramcontent.com/pod-product-compliance
Lightning Source LLC
Chambersburg PA
CBHW030529210326
41597CB00013B/1087